PRIMARY CONCERNS

By Sherry Ferrell

First printing February 2006

Disclaimer: This book is not written to give medical advice. For any advice you need concerning health problems you should consult your personal health care provider.

Table of Contents

For Pete, Chris, Sarah, and Shannon, with all my love.

Mom

Thank-you To all of my friends and family, and special thanks to Hanover Writers of Mechanicsville for your continual encouragement and support, my first writing experience has been very rewarding.

Forward

In the not too distant past good health was a natural by-product of just living. Today we must be vigilant to guard against adopting common practices that produce unhealthy results.

Modern technology has increased our lifespan and improved the quality of our lives in countless ways. On the same token our food supply has been changed affecting our ability to maintain good health.

Many of the foods we rely on have been altered from their natural state and contain substances that contribute to poor health.

Grains have been hybridized changing their beneficial qualities and currently the way some grains are harvested and stored; subtly invasive hidden mycotoxins are introduced that create the need for antibiotics that create health problems of their own.

The natural composition of dairy products and meats has been distorted by modern feeding practices producing foods that are laced with residues of antibiotics, growth hormone, and altered essential fatty acids.

Obtaining the ultimate texture and flavor has taken precedence over healthy goodness.

We have no idea that we are trading our health for convenience or simple pleasure. When we are faced with poor health as a result of adopting an ordinary lifestyle we have no idea how it happened or what to do about it.

Following is my story and approach to better health.

Words of Wisdom

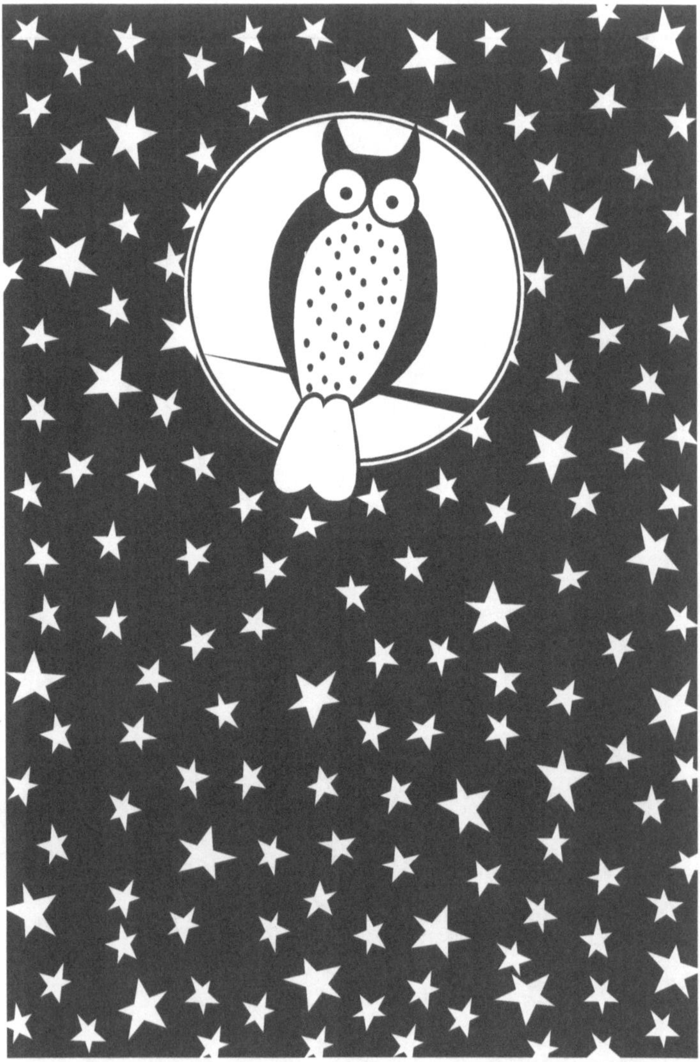

WORDS OF WISDOM

I am an ordinary person, a wife, mother, and friend.

After years of enduring recurring physical ailments I was led to research and experiment with the healing arts and discover the benefits of traditional healing techniques that are centuries old.

As I applied what I was learning I realized that wellness is more than the absence of disease and lifestyle affects health more than any other factor that might be considered.

The common practice of replacing healthy foods with foods that contribute to poor health is so overlooked that it is accepted as normal and has become customary.

Unhealthy foods are widely available because they cost less to produce so they have become pervasive.

Common ingredients in food are known to cause many health problems from lethargy and sugar cravings to diabetes and heart disease. Lack of fiber and nutrients, too much sugar, and the wrong kinds of fats are a natural by product of adopting an ordinary lifestyle. Most of us are so accustomed to this accepted way of life that we can't understand why we feel unwell.

Of all the healing modalities I tried during my struggle to achieve wellness, lifestyle had the greatest over-all effect on my physical condition.

It could not be disputed that pure water, clean air, and fresh foods are essential for total wellness and I discovered that the foundation of health is based upon the things we put on or into our bodies.

I also learned that healthy foods support the body in its ability to heal itself and provide energy and vitality. The right kinds of fats and sweeteners lower cholesterol and support cardiovascular health. Fresh meats oxygenate red blood cells and build muscle tissue. Fresh vegetables provide nutrients and fiber that help to regulate the bowels. Fresh fruits are natures candy and provide healthy goodness while satisfying our desire for sweets.

As I experimented with healthy diets I found that a one size fits all approach to lifestyle doesn't work for everyone. Each of us has special needs and our own bodies are the best indicator of what works for us and what does not.

As I strived to achieve a healthy lifestyle and find what worked for me I struggled with my lack of knowledge and my own ability to attain a healthy body.

The conditions that persisted in bothering me were of little concern to the health professionals who blithely wrote prescriptions for me, but never addressed the actual cause of my concerns as they sent me out the door.

As my awareness increased I longed for a medical practitioner with alternative wisdom to address my concerns. I had researched and accepted time-honored alternatives to conventional medicine and trusted those modalities, but I had not yet grown completely comfortable using the healing arts without assistance. I felt trapped into accepting conventional medical practices that were not helping, partly because I was insecure in my newfound health knowledge and also because my HMO paid for allopathic *(the treatment of a disease by using remedies whose effects differ from those produced by that disease)* medicine.

As I adopted a healthy lifestyle I continued to research and discovered a common factor in each of the conditions I was being treated for, which gave me hope that my ailments could be resolved. When I related my discovery to my primary care physician he scoffed and used a different approach to address my concerns. Feeling intimidated I dropped my query and continued my research until I became determined to get a referral to the correct health specialist.

Instead of getting the referral I had hoped for I got some unkindly offered "words of wisdom" from my primary care physician to the effect that my concerns were psychological.

His callous words forced me to accept the fact that I had to take total responsibility for my own health whether I was comfortable with the idea or not.

I reflected at length on how I had arrived at such a miserable impasse.

BLIND TRUST

BLIND TRUST

I had always lived in physical discomfort and had no idea that upper and lower abdominal pain, constipation, gas, bloating, indigestion and joint pain and stiffness were indicators of poor health. I grew up ignoring my physical symptoms.

At the age of twenty-one I left my home in Maine and moved to Florida, where I got a job at a truck stop restaurant working as a waitress.

When itchy coin shaped patches of skin began to develop on my forearms I thought it was from the detergent the restaurant used for cleaning the tables.

Over time diarrhea, chronic debilitating headaches that did not respond to analgesics and recurrent canker sores followed. It wasn't long before I exhibited a full-blown case of ulcerative colitis, was consequently hospitalized, lost time from work, and fired from my job.

More health problems followed and regular employment was nearly impossible.

I was evicted from my apartment and through some friends I found a rental property that needed fixing up. The first three months of rent and security deposit were waived in exchange for cleaning the place up and making minor repairs.

The property owner lived next door and operated a citrus stand that sold and shipped fresh oranges and grapefruits. She offered me a job and we worked together picking fruit and packing gift boxes for shipping.

For breakfast and snacks every day I ate fresh fruit. For lunch and supper I enjoyed Macdonald's or Wendy's hamburgers or Chinese take out.

The upper and lower abdominal discomfort I had always lived with turned to varying pains. Canker sores lined my top and bottom gum line and the back of my throat. My mouth was so sore I could barely eat anything. I began to experience frequent ear infections. My general practitioner said he usually saw those symptoms in small children.

Later when he cauterized the canker sores in my mouth for the third time in as many weeks he bluntly suggested I eat more oranges. After giving up citrus for a couple of weeks I discovered the elimination of oranges had no effect.

At times my head pounded for three days in a row and neither the analgesics I took nor the prescription my doctor had given me worked.

After a few more months of frequent doctor visits I could no longer afford treatment and I felt as though my doctor wanted to avoid seeing me. Since nothing was being resolved anyhow, I decided to stop seeking relief and just live with my symptoms.

I decided to leave sunny Florida and moved to Virginia where I met my husband.

When I was twenty-seven I had a severe toothache, and was hospitalized ten days for complications that arose after a dentist pulled the tooth even though it was abscessed, and the pharmacy forgot to tell me to take food with the prescription he'd given.

At twenty-nine my husband and I changed our health coverage to an HMO and selected an in-network healthcare provider.

I still lived with recurrent ailments so once again seeking relief, I made an appointment for the headaches, but the prescription I was given failed to affect the symptoms. The medicine for the canker sores was gross and ineffective. Exams for abdominal pain and discomfort revealed no causes.

My ankles had bothered me for years and were becoming increasingly painful. Upon examining my ankles my new doctor said the cartilage was completely gone and concluded that my pain would be permanent "because they didn't do ankle joint replacement yet".

He prescribed four buffered aspirin four times a day and suggested I wear ace bandages for support.

The pain in my ankles became so severe I crawled on my hands and knees to get up the stairs in our townhouse. At night I slept with my feet in a three-sided cardboard box to keep the blankets off of them.

The following year I was injured in a head on collision.

While my primary care physician was examining me, he suddenly jerked my head giving me the sensation of having been plugged into an electrical outlet, which was quickly followed by extreme pain.

I don't remember leaving the office or getting into my car. All I remember is feeling weak, nauseous and sweaty, and looking down at my itching feet discovering I had poison ivy. I must have walked through it when I got out of my car after the accident.

I sat in my car for a while and pulled myself together then went to the pharmacy to buy a bottle of calamine lotion before driving home. *(Since then I have learned about several homeopathic remedies that are symptom specific for poison ivy).*

When a friend phoned to see how I was doing I told her what was happening and she referred me to her chiropractor.

I was hesitant to see a chiropractor so I phoned the National Chiropractic Association asking for information regarding chiropractic care. The brochure I received helped to allay my fears.

Making that appointment turned out to be one of the best decisions I have ever made.

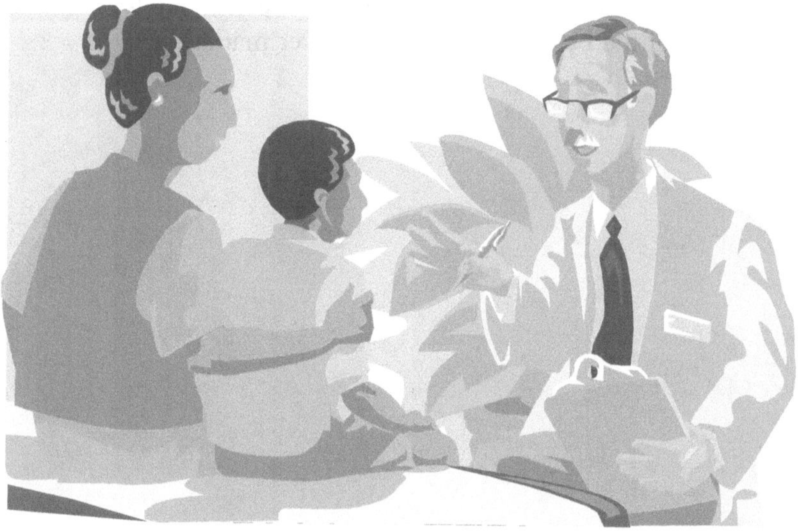

DOC C

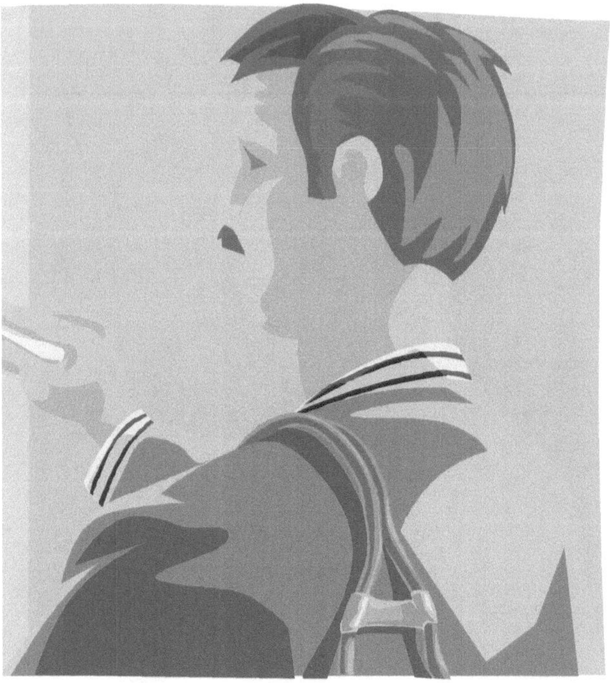

DOC C

The quality care I received from Doc "C" exceeded my expectations. He was pleasant and concerned. He took x-rays and told me about what he planned to do and why he would do it. He hooked me up to a wonderful machine that sent small pulses of electricity to my aching muscles, easing my pain. When my response to his question "when was your last bowel movement?" was "ten days ago," he showed alarm and told me I was being poisoned. He instructed me to drink a glass of orange juice well mixed with vegetable oil as soon as I got home.

He supplied me with a special pillow for my neck, a bottle of natural muscle relaxers and a topical preparation to rub into my aching muscles. As I was leaving his office he reminded me to see him again in three days.

When I got home not having any orange juice I mixed Doc C's recommended concoction with Kool-Aid. Good results were produced within twenty minutes.

During my next office visit Doc C let me know how serious my injuries were and informed me it would be at least three months before I could return to work.

For health insurance purposes I selected a new primary care physician who referred me to an orthopedist, who wrote me prescription medications for inflammation and pain and sent me on my way.

I continued to visit Doc C for chiropractic care and through his encouragement and generosity, borrowed some of his books on natural healing. I went home and began to read about natural healing and healthy living.

After I'd returned to work my ankles had become so inflamed it was becoming difficult to function.

Doc C did acupuncture, and I never required aspirin or ace bandages again because the pain was completely gone.

A few months later my husband and I decided to move from our townhouse to the family farm. I selected an in network health care provider in that area and began seeing him for frequent bouts of joint pain, muscle pain and stiffness, and periodic episodes of upper chest and back pain. After developing eczema on the entire back of my scalp and along the hairline on both sides of my head I became discouraged and dissatisfied.

I felt like my doctor didn't take me seriously and my symptoms continued to mount so I changed primary care physicians again.

One day after an appointment with Doc C as I was preparing to leave his office he said *"you keep digging around and someday somebody's really going to find something wrong with you and then where will you be"?* At first I was taken aback by his obtuse remark and felt like he didn't believe my symptoms were real either. But I knew Doc C had my best interests at heart or he wouldn't have given me food for thought.

While conventional medical care was less than ideal, HMO's did not cover Chiropractic or Naturopathic Doctors, and finding an M.D. who advocated natural healing would be like finding a needle in a haystack. I went out the door imagining what it would be like when "somebody" really resolved the many chronic ailments for which I relentlessly sought a solution.

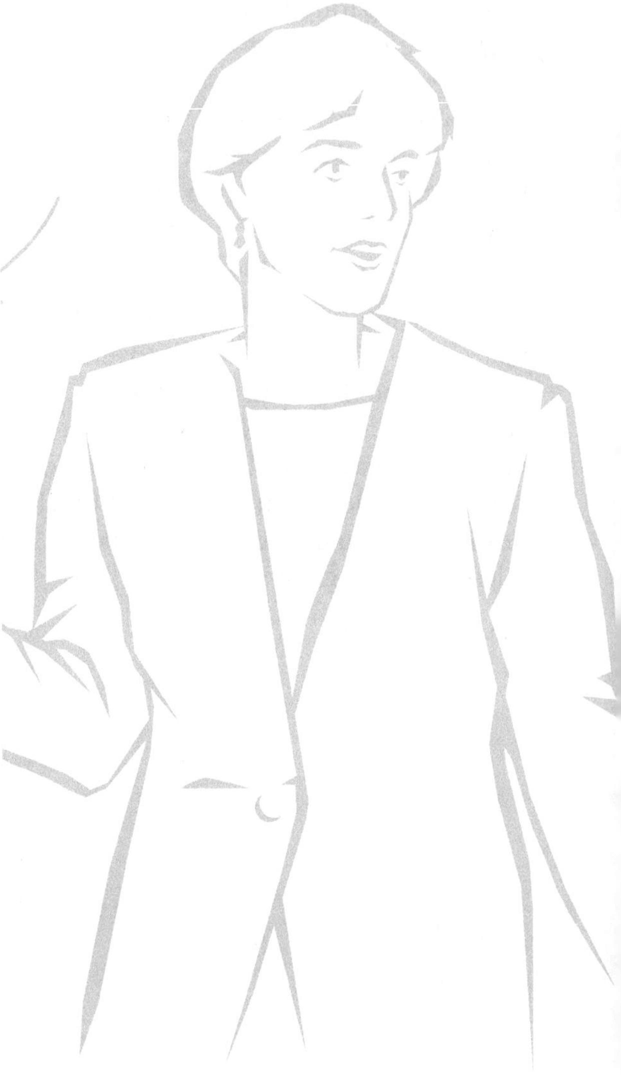

CONTEMPLATION

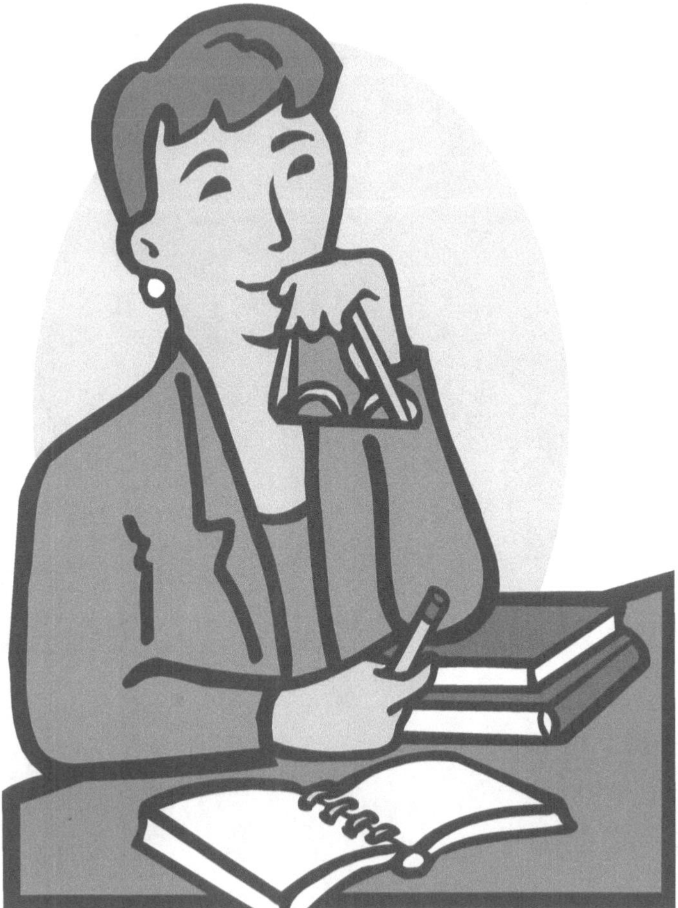

CONTEMPLATION

As time went by I wondered why my muscles and joints still hurt. When I could afford it I would make an appointment with Doc C to get some temporary relief from some of my symptoms and perhaps a little encouragement. I followed his suggestion to swim two or three days each week because it was easy on the joints, and I noticed some improvement in my mobility.

I continued to study natural healing and began learning about whole foods nutrition. I learned about the dangers of refined foods and how junk foods rob the body of vital nutrients *(for more information see the Choices P99-118).* I began making choices to improve the quality of my life.

I bought some whole foods cookbooks and experimented with the recipes.

When shopping for groceries instead of buying canned goods I bought fresh or frozen vegetables, and fruits.

When buying yogurt I looked for products with live active cultures of bifidophilus bacteria and avoided products with high fructose corn syrup or artificial sweeteners. Whenever possible I bought organic. The organic yogurt with cream on top was extraordinary!

I replaced margarines made from hydrogenated fat with real butter, flax seed oil, and olive oil, and replaced commercial peanut butter *(which is high in sugar, contains hydrogenated fat, and molds known as aflatoxins; suspected carcinogens)* with roasted almond butter.

I learned about sprouting grains to increase their nutritional content and bought whole-wheat and spelt berries and sprouted them. They had a sweet juicy crunch and were good added to salads and for snacks *(For more information on sprouting see*

P 166).

I bought and learned to cook with other whole grains like millet, amaranth, cracked wheat, bulgur, buckwheat, quinoa (pronounced keen-wah), and spelt. (P 163-164)

I added tofu (*bean curd*) and tempeh (*cultured bean curd*) and leaned heavily on whole grains and vegetables.

Sometimes I would make a large batch of oatmeal cookies for breakfasts or snacks.

It had been three years since the accident and I still endured the same old ailments. When my frustration level peaked I would go to my family doctor for relief, which proved to be symptomatic and temporary.

I developed jaw and face pain that my primary care physician diagnosed as TMJ or temporomandibular joint syndrome. He referred me to my dentist who fitted me for a plastic guard to wear over my teeth.

During follow up, my primary care physician prescribed anti-depressants, which caused constipation and cottonmouth.

I have since learned that Bach flower essences are a safe effective alternative to anti-depressants.

I bought a physician's desk reference so I could make informed decisions concerning the medications I was being prescribed. I learned to be cautious with Aspirin and Non-Steroidal Anti-inflammatory drugs because of my history with ulcerative colitis and ulcers.

Two more years passed and my ailments continued to bother me. Wanting a real solution for my problems I researched each condition I was being treated for.

As my knowledge increased I suspected food intolerance as the underlying cause of my symptoms. With that in mind I made an appointment with my primary care physician to get a referral to an allergist.

My primary care physician (of about three

years) scoffed at the idea and sent me to a gastroenterologist who during my initial consultation diagnosed me with irritable bowel syndrome, wrote me prescriptions for a powerful anti-spasmodic to control the symptoms and an anti-depressant to keep me from feeling bothered by my symptoms and sent me on my way.

My research showed me that most physicians consider IBS a psycho physiological disorder. Information showed that by a ratio of three to one women are more commonly affected than men and the cause is considered to be stress related. A normal diet is recommended; if constipation or spastic colon is present an increase in dietary fiber is advised.

Common illnesses that may be confused with IBS are lactose intolerance, and allergic gastroenteropathy (Merck Manual of Diagnosis and Therapy).

I was disappointed with the diagnosis the gastroenterologist had given me and disliked being considered neurotic. When I looked up the prescribed medicines in the physician's desk reference and noted the side effects, I decided not to get them filled. I knew there had to be a way to determine the cause and address it.

During my follow up appointment with my primary care physician he advised me to use Metamucil to increase the amount of fiber in my diet. The results of doing as he suggested were disastrous in that it plugged up my bowels and caused uncontrollable leaking of fluid around the hardened fecal matter.

Fresh fruits and vegetables are high in fiber especially when raw. Salads are an excellent way to enjoy raw fruits and vegetables.

I discontinued the fiber supplements.

Researching gave me hope that something would get resolved so I kept studying natural healing guides as well as conventional healing guides. I discovered that all of my symptoms and diagnosed conditions could be found in conjunction with food allergy and intolerance. I began to see that food allergy and intolerance and most of the conditions associated with them are also diagnosed as psycho physiological disorders.

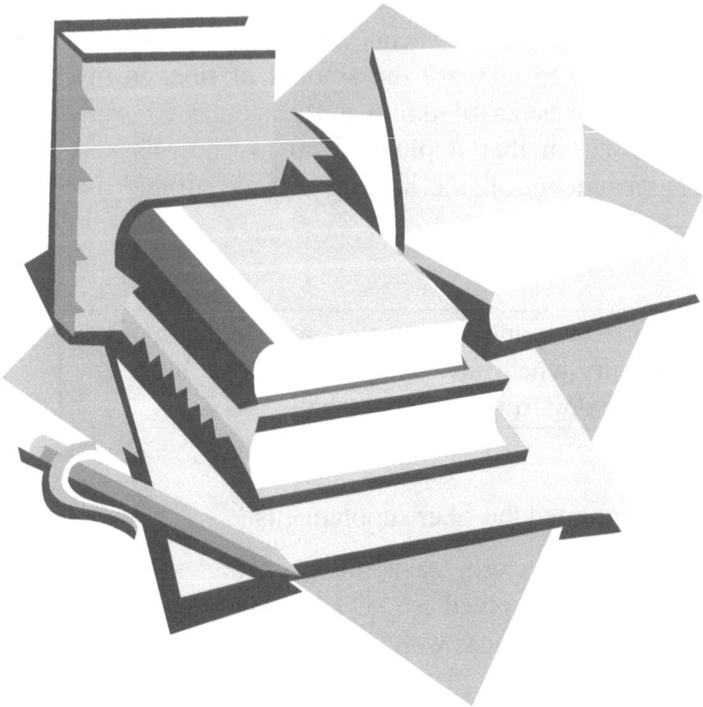

THE CATALYST

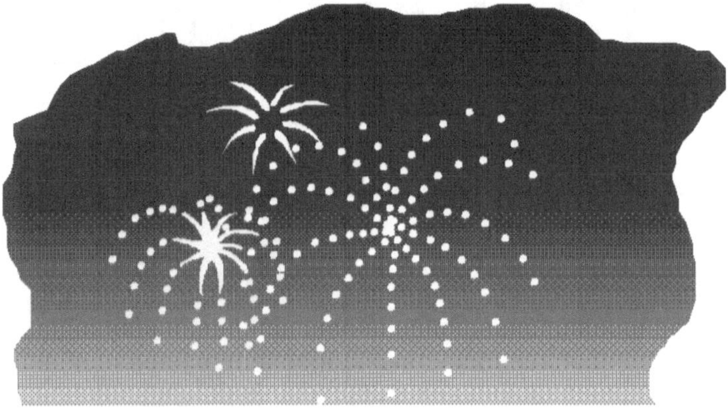

THE CATALYST

It had been five years since the accident and fifteen years since the beginning of my ailments. I had grown increasingly uncomfortable in my own body and had become totally disappointed and completely frustrated with the quality of healthcare I was receiving.

I fully realized the drawbacks of using prescription medications that suppressed symptoms instead of addressing the original causes, and I finally understood that most medical doctors used set procedures that rarely differed from one practitioner to another.

Since medical doctors all used the same standard procedures to address symptoms it seemed useless to seek another, so I stuck with the one I was seeing at that time and continued to do my own research. I came to the conclusion that prescription medicines were not going to help me resolve anything.

Resolving my discomfort became a driving force in my life. I wanted a real solution for my problems and became more determined than ever to rid myself of the many chronic conditions that were continuing to mount.

Because nothing had been resolved and the

side effects from the prescriptions I was taking were adding to my discomfort instead of alleviating it I decided to discontinue all the medications I was taking including the anti-depressants slowly weaning myself off of them because research revealed stopping them suddenly was not advised.

I was studying herbal healing and planned on using herbs after I learned more about them when a new symptom surfaced. This time it was rectal bleeding.

Once again I visited my primary care physician.

He examined me and diagnosed the condition as hemorrhoids, then gave me a preparation in a tube, instructed me in its use, and sent me on my way.

Having had hemorrhoids, I wasn't convinced that was the cause of my problem and decided against the use of the hemorrhoid preparation.

When the symptoms persisted, I was scheduled for an in office sigmoid colonoscopy.

During the procedure it was discovered that the equipment was clogged from previous use on other patients.

I was horrified and in complete shock!

The doctor stopped the examination and took the scope over to a large sink in the corner of the room where he and his nurse scrubbed it with hot soapy water.

Still lying on the examination table I looked over in disbelief while they worked to correct the problem.

Stunned, shaken, and totally disgusted I had no idea what I should do. My heart pounded and my mind raced!

A sickening feeling washed over me. “Maybe I should get up and walk out”?

I thought about the health problems I had experienced over the years leading up to that moment. The conditions that had persisted in bothering me had been nuisance ailments and I felt like a nuisance myself. I thought, “Maybe I’m a hypochondriac after all. But I don’t think you can imagine rectal bleeding. If I hadn’t persisted in finding a solution to my ailments I wouldn’t be in this predicament”.

I recalled Doc C’s obtuse remark and realized he’d been right all along. I wavered between walking out and finishing the procedure. I had gone through a lot to prepare for this exam. If I got up and walked out I would have to find another doctor who would recommend the same approach. The preparation for this examination was disgusting and I didn't want to have to go through that again!

I felt trapped between a rock and a hard place. I figured it was too late to worry about what I might have been exposed to so I made the decision to stay and finish the procedure.

As soon as it was over I hurried to the bathroom, jumped up and down to get the air out of my colon, washed up, got dressed, and headed for the exit.

As soon as my husband and I got in the car to go home I blurted out the whole experience. We rode home in stunned silence.

For days afterward I worried about what I might have been exposed to. Finally I decided to push it out of my mind. It was water over the dam now.

A few days later my doctor informed me that no abnormalities were found and he set up an appointment for me *(which he should have done to begin with*) with a proctologist.

During my appointment with the proctologist I learned that the in office procedure with my primary care physician had been completely unnecessary and the two conditions that were noted by the specialist and his nurse on visual exam required surgery. He diagnosed my symptoms as an anal fissure and a fistula and strongly advised me against the use of hemorrhoid preparations. He also informed me I should call immediately if I experienced any pain or spasms and then scheduled me for surgery.

When I got home I researched the two diagnosed conditions and found they were caused by chronic constipation *(I assumed from the prescription medications I had been taking).* I looked up herbs for pain associated with constipation and noted some common ingredients that might prove helpful. Among them was the ordinary kitchen spice ginger. Later I found a box of ginger tea at the health food store and tried it. It was warming and had a pleasant taste when I added a spoonful of honey *(I have since learned to make my tea with fresh ginger, which is more effective than dried ginger P 198).*

The week before the surgery my mother came down from Maine for a visit. I had wanted to ride the Jamestown Ferry, and, since Jamestown was less than an hours drive from the house we decided to go. Mom and I headed out right after breakfast.

We had ridden the ferry across the James River and were on our way toward Chippokes plantation. I was driving when the spasm hit. I pulled over and parked on the side of the road. My mother got behind the wheel and drove until she found a recreation center where they had a bathroom.

I entered the building and found myself in a large gymnasium where some teenagers were playing basketball. I looked around for a bathroom, noting it was on the other side of the basketball court.

I made my way to the facility and chose the handicapped stall thankful for the bars that were built in for support. Sweating profusely and gripped with pain I removed my shirt and pants and sat on the toilet. After several ineffectual minutes I put my shirt back on, pulled myself up and finished dressing.

When I got out to the car I crawled into the back seat and curled up as much as the space would allow. Lying in the back seat of the car as my mother drove I gave her directions to get us back home.

At home I phoned the proctologist and was instructed to fill the bathtub with hot water to ease the spasms.

My mother made me a cup of hot ginger tea sweetened with honey while I filled the bathtub with hot water.

I took huge swallows of the tea to help alleviate the pain. (*I chose ginger over an ordinary pain reliever because it was symptom specific*). While I soaked in the tub I thought about my remedy selection wondering if it was correct. It seemed to help at any rate.

Later, research showed that I had chosen correctly.

Ginger is effective for relieving many symptoms including inflammation and pain especially spasms associated with constipation.

The morning of the surgery I woke up with a cold so I called the surgeon who advised I have a local anesthetic and I should just mention that he said so.

While I was being prepped for the surgery I reminded the nurse that I had a cold, was getting a local anesthetic and gave the name of my doctor.

I was given injections through my IV that I later found were for general anesthesia. I was awake during the procedure but heavily drugged.

After the surgery I got very sick and every few minutes the anesthesiologist would walk by and say in broken English "I no make you sick". Finally my nurse sternly told him not to come back.

I had been admitted early that morning for surgery as an outpatient but because I was sick for so long I was admitted to a regular room in the hospital. I went home late that evening.

Two weeks after my surgery I saw the proctologist for a follow up visit and was referred back to my primary care physician.

After the experience during the in office colonoscopy my respect for my primary care physician was gone. I knew other doctors used the same approaches to healing that he did and I had little hope of finding anyone better. I decided to keep seeing him even though he was less than ideal, but only if there was a pressing need.

I wondered if our HMO was a factor in the quality of my healthcare or the reason why in-network healthcare providers seemed to be poured from the same mold.

When my ears stopped up, started ringing, and I couldn't get my balance, I made an appointment with a physician out of network hoping to have a different experience. He gave me a sample medication with no explanation for my problem and sent me on my way. I paid him out of pocket, went home, looked the medication up in the physician's desk reference and noted that it was an anti-histamine. I took it realizing I could get some over the counter if I needed it again. I also realized that the underlying cause of my headaches was allergies.

It was now seven years since the accident

and two years since the surgery.

I was experiencing all of my old ailments and now tender points and sharp aching pains on various parts of my body. All of my joints ached and were slightly swollen. I was also physically exhausted.

I was fully aware that medical doctors addressed symptoms not causes. I wanted to switch to a Naturopathic doctor, but was paying for an HMO so I couldn't afford one.

I was convinced I had food intolerance, and I was determined to get a referral to an allergist. I called my doctor's office and made an appointment.

When my doctor entered the examination room I was waiting in he sat down in front of me and leaned over real close to my face. I could feel his warm breath on the side of my face and neck as he leaned toward my ear and quietly said, "There are more important things to do in this world than to feel sorry for yourself".

" OH REALLY," I thought considering where these valuable words of wisdom were coming from.

From the same doctor whom about two years previously during an unnecessary in office sigmoid colonoscopy had informed his assistant that the medical device they had inserted fully into my colon was clogged from previous use on others.

Disgusted! Certainly! But definitely not “sorry” for myself!

The only thing I was feeling sorry for was sticking with this abject practitioner out of sheer desperation to resolve the chronic conditions that persisted to bother me!

Inwardly seething, I drove home contemplating how many other physicians there are cut from the same cloth. I should know! I think I’ve seen them all!

He was just like every other conventional medical practitioner I had seen over the years. He subjected me to the same prescriptions, procedures, protocol, and air of indifference I had come to expect.

Only instead of quietly projecting his opinion through body language, he had the audacity to reveal it!

My discomfort, frustration, ignorance, and unrelenting determination to resolve my symptoms had brought me to this sorry state of affairs and I realized I’d finally wound up at the last resort.

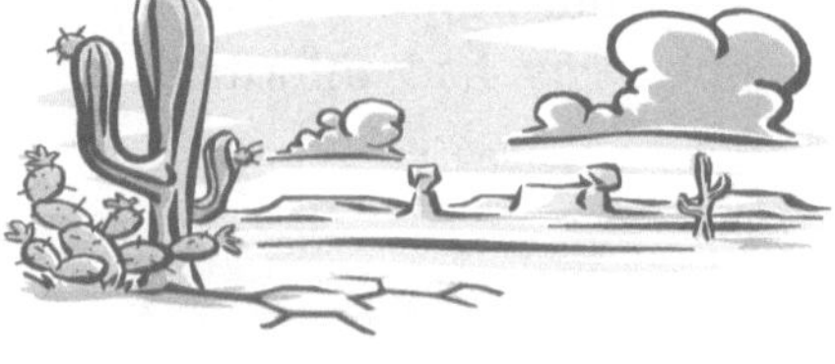

VERACITY

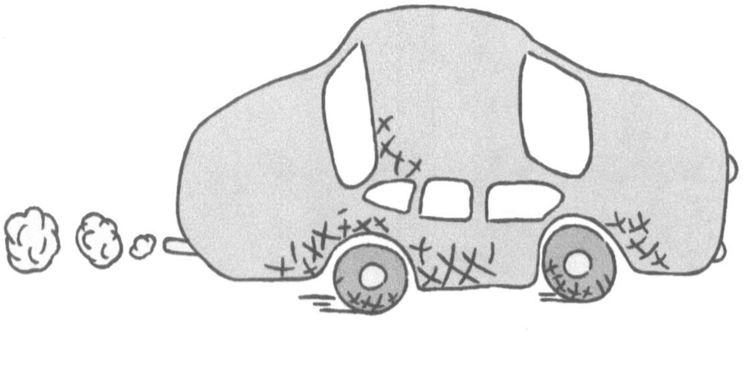

VERACITY

As I drove home I faced the fact that there wasn't a primary care physician or general practitioner anywhere who would ever use any other approach than the ones I had already suffered through for the last seventeen years.

Continuing to trudge endlessly from one primary care physician to another or wishing my health insurance paid for chiropractic care or naturopathic physicians was not going to solve any of my problems.

I had no other alternative than to solve my health problems on my own.

Armed with new determination I went home and called my doctor's office and told his receptionist I needed a referral from my insurance company and an appointment with an allergist.

I was pleasantly surprised when she followed through without question.

Allergy testing confirmed food allergies and intolerances as well as allergies to inhalants or environmental allergies.

Allergy shots for grasses, dust mites and mold were prescribed.

I was instructed to cover my pillow and mattress with slipcovers, read food labels, and avoid substances I was allergic or intolerant to;

especially soy, corn, beef, and milk, which showed the greatest reactions during testing. Tea, strawberries, citrus, mustard *(includes canola oil)*, kale, garlic, carrots, peanuts, chocolate, grapes, barley, malt and hops were to be avoided as well *(My allergies to grasses would prove to be my biggest concern*).

I was given an appointment with the nurse to learn how to give myself allergy shots and referred back to my primary care physician for follow up.

During the follow-up appointment my primary care physician told me *his sister had been getting allergy shots for years and had seen a reduction in her symptoms.* As he was saying that I recalled the time he had scoffed at the idea and informed me that there was no such a thing as allergies. I was glad I had decided not to see him anymore.

When I got home I sat down and wrote him a letter of appreciation thanking him for referring me to the allergist and for his *expertise* and *dedication* as a *medical professional.* I changed primary care physicians, vowing to be seen only for "conditions that are beyond my ability to care for myself".

I left my old records and chronic ailments behind.

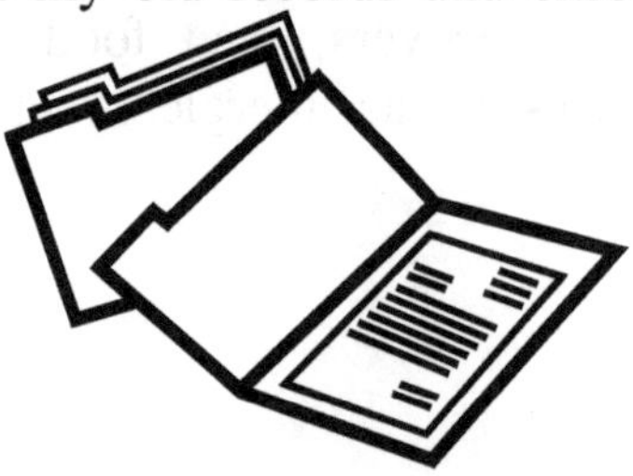

LEARNING PROCESS

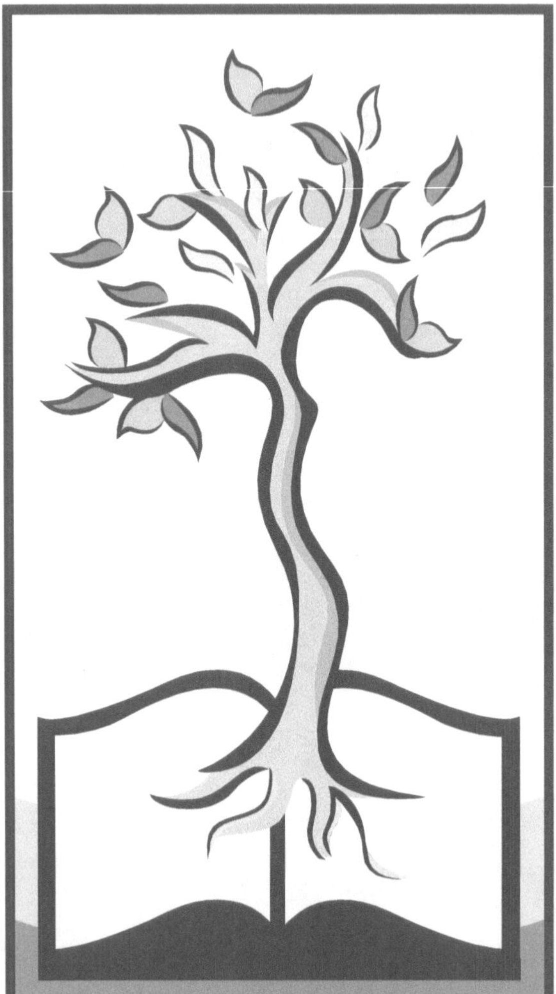

LEARNING PROCESS

Being tested for allergies, learning to read food labels, and avoiding the substances I was intolerant to improved the quality of my life and I was able to minimize the number of my health problems. But I had a lot to learn before all of them would be resolved.

As I eliminated and reintroduced foods, I became aware of the cause and effect of each of my symptoms.

Tea and grapes made me extremely tired.

Sometimes I broke out in hives when I ate strawberries.

Dairy products caused congestion and ringing ears.

Right sided lower abdominal pain, rectal pain, and canker sores were related to the consumption of beef.

Soy caused cramping, bloating, and excess gas.

Eating corn, rice, rye and chocolate caused a gradual buildup of sinus pressure and pounding headaches.

Barley caused rapid heartbeat and nervousness.

As I reduced my exposure to allergens my joint pains eased.

Finding cereals without corn, rice, or barley malt was very difficult. One hundred percent Shredded Wheat was all I could find. Soaked in hot water, or apple juice, it was pretty good.

I still lived with upper back and chest pain, some cramping, and bloating. Occasionally my lower back would go out for no apparent reason. *(Lower back pain later proved to be IBS)*

During the grass pollen season my sinuses would fill with fluid, causing dizziness, loss of balance and ringing ears.

The humidity in summer exacerbated my eczema and I rubbed the skin on my arms and legs raw from the constant itching.

The allergy shots caused repeated reactions so I discontinued them.

I collected resources on natural healing and continued my research on allergies and food intolerance.

Diversity

And then to my satisfaction I discovered I was pregnant and in the usual length of time I gave birth to a beautiful baby girl! I decided to breastfeed.

When my daughter was six-weeks old we moved because the house we were renting had been sold. While my husband was at work my fourteen year old son and I packed, loaded our pick-up truck, and made several trips to and from our new location about eight miles away. I snacked on oatmeal cookies while I was driving back and forth between houses. By the end of the day my baby girl had severe diarrhea. I took her to the pediatrician who admitted her to the hospital because of dehydration.

As soon as we got to the hospital we were sent directly to the pediatric floor, and given a room. The nurse acquainted us with our space, helped us get comfortable and left.

She came back soon and told us we would be going down the hall in a few minutes and she quietly suggested I insist on being present with my baby at all times.

A few minutes later we were led down the hall to a large room set up with lots of equipment for various procedures.

There were two women in the room who introduced themselves and informed me that they were resident doctors with the hospital. One of them took my daughter from my arms and laid her tiny body on a board with a nylon restraint and strapped her down "for her protection".

The other one told me they would get back to me in a few minutes.

When I insisted on staying with my baby they began to gather things up and put them away. I wondered what unnecessary procedures they had planned to practice on my daughter.

One of the women drew blood, while the other tried to insert a catheter and failed, much to my relief. *(I was concerned it would cause a bladder infection and feared it might puncture her bladder, which is not uncommon)* I could see a questioning terrified look in my baby girl's eyes and was unable to cuddle her so I held her little hand and reassured her that everything would be all right. A tiny IV was inserted in her leg and they sent us back to our room where my husband was waiting. I told him everything I had observed and suspected, thankful that I had insisted on being with our daughter at all times.

The next morning we all went home and I eliminated oats from our diet.

A few months later when we started our daughter on her first solid food, she vomited it back up. She was intolerant to rice. Her pediatrician assured me that breast-fed babies do not get allergies. She developed ear infections and exhibited intolerances to antibiotics and over the counter medicines. History was repeating itself.

Impart

Learning about healthy living became a passion. Anytime we had extra money we would go to the bookstore.

I was reading a book called The ABC Herbal: A Natural Health Guide for Children-- by Steven H. Horne that mentioned peeling and using fresh garlic for ear infections. I tried it for myself when my ears started ringing and it worked very well. I was delighted but my husband turned up his nose.

The book also mentioned taping a small slice of garlic to a sensitive area of the body first to see if the skin blisters, as some people are sensitive to garlic.

I have since learned that garlic can be used to remove warts by applying a slice to the surface of the wart with a band-aid and leaving it on for at least twenty-four hours. In a few days the wart usually falls off leaving a tiny crater and the skin gradually heals over the spot where the wart used to be.

Option

When I developed a raging bladder infection I thought about going to a doctor but it was the middle of the night and my husband and children were sleeping. The idea of waking my family to spend hours waiting in the emergency room deterred me. Remembering the two-hour rule I had discovered during research, I looked up herbal medicines for cystitis and selected Echinacea to try and ease my discomfort until morning when the doctor's office opened.

> For acute conditions herbal medicines can be taken every fifteen minutes for up to two hours.

I followed the recommended dosage and took two capsules every fifteen minutes for two hours. By the end of the two hours the pain was completely gone and I was my old self again.

To prevent a relapse I continued to take five hundred milligrams of echinacea three times a day for a total of seven days. (If you are sensitive to ragweed avoid Echinacea. The herb oregon grape has properties that are similar to those found in Echinacea).

Homeopathy

I had not researched or planned to use homeopathics.

I had seen references to the medicines in some of my books during research but being unfamiliar with the modality had considered the remedies to be rare or obscure.

My introduction to homeopathic medicines came about through trial and error when I bought a kit for children at an herb store mistaking it for herbs. It contained several remedies specific for teething, cuts, scrapes, bumps, bruises, and common ailments. The kit had been drastically reduced in price because the lid was cracked and it had a broken hinge. I bought it and when I got home I put it in the hall closet.

A few weeks later during the night our baby girl woke up screaming. Nothing we tried would console her.

I remembered the children's homeopathic remedy kit and went to the closet and took it out. It had a booklet in it that described the remedies, what they were for, and how to use them. Chamomilla was specific for a screaming child who could not be consoled. I opened the chamomilla bottle, followed the instructions and dumped one pill into the bottle cap as directed, being sure not to touch it. The instructions had said to take one tablet under the tongue and let it melt. I dropped the little powdery pill from the bottle cap directly under my daughters tongue and put the cap back on the bottle. By the time I got the kit back into the hall closet she had stopped screaming. At that moment I thought, " what a coincidence, she's stopped crying already", and went back to bed. *(Through research I later found that Chamomilla is not only calming but it also relieves pain associated with teething and other ailments)*

Another night I woke up in with a pounding headache. With hopes of avoiding antihistamines I got the homeopathic remedy kit out of the closet and looked up the remedies for headaches. Uncertain about which medicine to use I selected homeopathic belladonna, placed it under my tongue, put the kit away, and went back to bed. My pounding headache persisted and I began to feel very cold. I went back to the remedy kit, took out the booklet and looked at the information on belladonna again. One of the characteristics of the remedy was that it removes heat from the body. I put the booklet and kit away and considered the remedies. The kit did say homeopathic remedies not herbal remedies. I decided to find out more about homeopathic medicine.

The next day I bought a book called Homeopathic Medicine At Home by Maesimund B. Panos, M.D. and Jane Heimlich and discovered more about the wonders of homeopathy. The book listed many common ailments and remedy selections. It described the basic principles of homeopathy, how to use it effectively and the specifics of each remedy.

With the kids in tow I went back to the little herb store and bought a Hyland's 30x Homeopathic medicine kit that contained twenty-eight of the most commonly used remedies.

Later I bought the books Homeopathy for Pregnancy, Birth, and your Baby's first year by Miranda Castro, and The Consumer's Guide To Homeopathy The Definitive Resource for Understanding Homeopathic Medicine and Making It Work for You by Dana_Ullman, M. P. H. coauthor of Everybody's Guide to Homeopathic Medicine. As I applied this healing modality I found it practical and effective.

Homeopathic medicines have been used for more than two hundred years. They are symptom specific and very effective. Homeopathy can be applied for emotional as well as physical well-being.

There are specific guidelines that must be followed to ensure correct use. Once the basics are learned the medicines become practical for everyday concerns that might come up.

For the novice the X potencies like 12x or 30x are ideal as they wear off sooner than the C potencies like 6c or 30c so if the wrong remedy was selected the waiting time before making another selection is considerably shorter. Taken correctly homeopathic remedies can reduce duration time and ease symptoms. They are great to have on hand for self-limited conditions that usually go away on their own in a week to ten days.

For chronic conditions it is preferable to seek the assistance of a professional homeopath.

Over the years I have used these remedies for the needs of my self, my husband, children, pets, and farm animals. Used correctly they are very effective. Another plus is that they are also inexpensive.

It is very important to stop using any homeopathic remedy at the first sign of improvement.

When I first started using homeopathic remedies my daughter had a blocked tear duct in one of her eyes. The tear duct had been blocked since she was born and I feared surgery was imminent. I selected the correct remedy but failed to stop at the first sign of improvement, balance was exceeded and the blockage worsened. I kept giving the remedy as the condition worsened and it got really bad. I finally had to find a professional homeopath to help reverse the effects of my error. We were fortunate that she was easily able to do so and I learned a valuable lesson at my daughter's expense.

When using any remedy learn what you need it for, what it consists of, how safe it is, how effective it is, how to use it, and use it responsibly.

Learning about Fresh Juice and Grinding Grain

My sister phoned because our mother had been hospitalized and was seriously ill so my husband and I packed up the kids and the family car and we drove from our home in Virginia to Maine for a visit. She recovered well and we came back home.

During the drive back we stopped at a rest area on the Garden State Parkway just outside New York and I went inside to seek refreshment. I spotted a juice-bar and decided to try something. Waiting in line I looked over the menu and selected the Ginger-Hopper. It consisted of fresh ginger, carrots, and an apple.

The juice had a naturally sweet taste with a hint of ginger. I drank it while I was driving. It tasted great and I was perked up all the way to Delaware!

As soon as we got home I went shopping for a juicer. I bought a juice machine and the book Juicing for Life by Cherie Calbom and Maureen Keane and found out how to make my own Ginger-Hopper and many other refreshing juices.

Later I graduated to a champion juicer, added a grain mill to it, and started grinding organic wheat berries to make our own flour for whole grain wheat bread with all the healthy fiber, oils and nutrients still intact. I learned to make home milled cream of wheat cereal and other hot cereals from different grains like amaranth and buckwheat.

Enlightened

We got a computer and I went online to see if sugar cane was a grass. I spotted an article about sinus conditions related to grass pollen that suggested symptoms could be controlled by avoiding grains three months prior to the grass pollen season.

At that moment I realized why my ears were ringing and stopped up! And why I was dizzy during grass pollen season!

I had tested positive for environmental sensitivities to grass pollen and allergies to corn, barley, and malt. I suspected rice, rye, and oats.

Further research revealed all the substances included in the grass family. (GRAMINEAE)

BAMBOO SHOOTS, BARLEY, RYE, KAMUT, SPELT, TRITICALE, WHEAT, OATS, TEFF, RICE, WILD RICE, MILLET, MILO, MOLASSES, SORGHUM, SUGAR CANE, CANE SUGAR, AND CORN. (I later discovered that the herb lemongrass is also in the grass family of plants).

So I cleaned out the pantry and threw out all the cereals, grains and sweeteners. Because sensitivities to wheat had not shown up during allergy testing and no obvious symptoms were noted I decided not to eliminate wheat. (*I would eventually realize my mistake).*

Quinoa, amaranth, and buckwheat are not true grains as they are not plants belonging to the grass family so I kept them in our diet.

I replaced granulated white sugar with date sugar and bought bean-based pasta and buckwheat noodles (soba).

Goat's Milk

I wanted to own goats and had heard the milk was a good substitute for cows' milk. I became the proud owner of three beautiful milk does. During the following summer I looked like one big oozing rash and my ears were ringing. My daughter had some eczema now as well.

> Homeopathy is not recommended for eczema especially if it is chronic as eczema is an outward sign of a deeper problem.

We stopped using goats' milk and went back to cooking with non-dairy ingredients and having our cereal with water or apple juice. Our eczema cleared up and the goats became family pets.

Course of Action

As time passed my upper chest and back pain became more pronounced. My face grew round and my skin gradually turned yellow.

I developed a brownish patch of discoloration on my upper left cheek and began to experience shortness of breath and dizzy spells.

A visit to the emergency room revealed gallstones.

The diagnosis was made by a nurse who laughingly recited a poem to me, saying, "female, fair, fat and forty, it must be gallstones"!

Needless to say I was not amused. (*Especially considering I had exhibited the symptoms for more than twenty years*).

I was sent to radiology, the stones were confirmed, and surgery was recommended.

When the surgeon I visited described the

surgery to me, I asked him about alternatives. He told me surgery was the only alternative. I decided not to have the surgery. He said, "You'll be back". I thought, “Not if I can help it”.

I tried a raw vegetable juice fast for a few days and went to see a local herbalist who advised a gallbladder flush.

I went home and consulted some reference materials, which noted a gallbladder flush was <u>not</u> advised if you had cholecystitis *(inflammation of the gallbladder),* tried it anyways and understood why it was a bad idea.

The night of the gallbladder flush the pain was so severe the next day I went back to the surgeon’s office and asked for the surgery. I had my gallbladder removed two days later learning my gallstones were extremely large.

After the surgery I thought that the upper back and chest pain would go away but it didn’t.

Trials

Time passed and wanting to lose weight I decided to try a low carbohydrate diet. I looked at the different plans and chose the Atkins diet. After trying the diet for a few weeks, eliminating sugars and starches, then introducing them back into my diet I noticed starchy foods disagreed with me. I went online and typed in a search for starches and

IBS. I hit the super highway jackpot of information!

A website called The Healing Crow (www.healingcrow.com) appeared with information about non-drug related approaches to healing chronic illnesses. I clicked on ***Our Story*** and read Seth Barrows account of his trials with crohn's disease and noted his mention of a book, which details a specific carbohydrate diet for healing intestinal disorders. The book BREAKING THE VICIOUS CYCLE: Intestinal Health Through Diet By Elaine Gottschall B.A.,M.Sc. has helped many people with crohn's disease and ulcerative colitis to become symptom free. As stated on the healing crow website, today, the SCD is being used successfully by many to treat the following: Autism, Crohn's disease, Ulcerative Colitis, Celiac disease, Cystic Fibrosis, Chronic Diarrhea, Candidiasis, and Irritable Bowel Syndrome (IBS). I clicked on the link (www.scdiet.org) to the web site for The Specific Carbohydrate Diet, then clicked on another link for the book. Not wanting to wait to read the book I found a copy at a local bookstore.

There were recipes in the book and on the website. They were plentiful and varied so I tried the diet for several weeks. I learned about almond flour to replace wheat flour and other grains. Why honey is preferred as a sweetener, how to make a special yogurt that was free of lactose (the sugar in milk) and the availability of lactose free cheeses.

I knew I was intolerant to dairy but I was hoping the removal of lactose would make a difference. So I tried the diet for a few weeks, tweaking the baked goods recipes to make the texture and flavor more to my liking.

My eczema increased and my ears started ringing.

I went back online and did a new search on starches and IBS, found the link to The Healing Crow and read their comments on The Paleo Diet a stricter diet than the Specific Carbohydrate Diet.

Recipes are available @www.paleofood.com and information about what the hunter/gatherers ate @ www.paleodiet.com.

The Paleo diet is grain-free, bean-free, potato-free, dairy-free and sugar-free.

INGREDIENTS USED ARE: meat, fish, poultry, vegetables, fruits, nuts, seeds, berries and honey. Fats from meat, coconuts, and olives are used.

I bought the books The Paleo Diet: Lose Weight and Get Healthy By Eating The Foods You Were Designed To Eat—by Loren Cordain and Neanderthin: Eat Like A Caveman to Achieve a Lean, Strong Healthy Body-- by Ray Audette who has used this way of eating to reverse the progression of arthritis and diabetes.

I started the paleo diet and applied most of what I had learned from the specific carbohydrate diet deciding not to use the recommended fats suggested and used butter instead.

It was a decision I would come to regret.

My eczema cleared up and I experienced upper chest and back pain that felt like gallbladder pain. Since I no longer had a gallbladder I became confused and panicked.

My primary care physician was no longer participating with my health insurance company. I saw my new primary care physician and was diagnosed with ulcers. I disagreed because the pain felt similar to gallstones but he wouldn't budge. He gave me a prescription to reduce stomach acid and sent me on my way.

I went home and researched to learn as much as possible about ulcers and the recommended treatment.

My new primary care physician had not tested for H. Pylori.

> H. Pylori or Helicobacter Pylori is a bacterium that is often present with stomach ulcers.

In the absence of testing for H. Pylori I

decided not to take the prescription to reduce stomach acid when there was no indication of an over acid condition.

Reducing stomach acid unnecessarily can impair digestion and mock acid reflux disease (P121).

After researching and viewing many separate articles on ulcers and herbal treatment options I decided to use herbs that were proven effective for healing ulcers and bismuth (*Pepto-Bismol*) to destroy the bacteria. I chose Licorice Root, which soothes inflammation and protects the stomach from the effects of stomach acid. Because I was planning to use licorice for more than seven days I used DGL Licorice that has been processed to remove the compound that raises blood pressure. (DGL is the abbreviation for deglycyrrhizinated).

A couple of days later I became alarmed because my stools had turned black and I made an appointment with the nurse practitioner to ensure nothing was seriously wrong with me.

I was informed that black stools were a common side effect from taking bismuth. I asked for a test to confirm the presence of H. Pylori bacteria. It came back negative.

When I got home I got out a magnifying glass and looked on the back of the bottle of bismuth and saw in really fine print, *this beneficial medication may cause temporary and harmless darkening of the tongue or stool.*

After two weeks when the pain was unresolved I scheduled another appointment with the nurse practitioner. All I got was the feeling I was being brushed off.

More research revealed that my symptoms mimicked a condition usually seen in cases of severe alcoholism.

A few months later I experienced an attack that was so painful I doubled over and started sweating. My stools were a much lighter color and spongy looking. I scheduled an immediate appointment with the nurse practitioner and stressed the fact that I was very health conscious and was concerned about the symptoms I was observing. She ordered lab work and decided to send me to a gastroenterologist for testing.

The gastroenterologist told me after I described my symptoms that I had functional IBS and handed me prescriptions for antidepressants and antispasmodics informing me I must take them or I could not be helped. Appointments for radiological exams of my upper and lower digestive system and an endoscopy and colonoscopy were scheduled. I decided to wait to fill the prescriptions until after testing was completed because the side effects were risky.

When the radiological exams showed no abnormalities I decided to cancel the appointments for the endoscopy and colonoscopy. A couple of weeks later the upper chest and back pain increased again so I rescheduled the appointments for the tests.

During the fast the night before the endoscopy and colonoscopy I noticed that the upper back and chest pain were completely gone.

With that in mind, after the procedure I started to examine my diet closely. The only thing left to consider eliminating from my diet was butter. I researched and found information showing that my symptoms were related to lactose intolerance and undigested fats. I discontinued using butter and increased my use of extra virgin olive oil. The upper back and chest pain cleared up and my stools returned to a non-spongy more colored state. Since then I have found that when I eat grains I have excess gas, feel bloated, and my stools are less frequent (several days), larger, darker, and more difficult to pass. While on the paleo diet the stools are more frequent (daily) lighter in color, smaller, and much easier to pass.

I went back to the gastroenterologist for the follow up appointment and was informed that the procedures showed no abnormalities or obvious causes for my discomfort.

Attainment

Feeling better I continued with the Paleo diet. In my opinion it is whole foods nutrition at it's best. It eliminates most of my problem foods and my family enjoys the recipes as much as I do. There aren't any overpriced, expensive, strange, or unusual foods on this plan. And everything needed is available from my local grocery store.

(Grass fed meat is optimal for this diet as grain fed meat, is high in omega-6 fatty acids and retains residues of growth hormone and antibiotics. If grass fed meat is not feasible taking omega-3 fish oil supplements to offset the high omega-6 content of commercially raised animal products is recommended). *(omega-3 fats p101-102)*

After giving up all grains and the goods derived from them such as breads cereals and desserts; all my aches and pains disappeared. I had more energy, my sinuses and skin completely cleared and my bowel movements were lighter in color, more frequent, smaller, and easier to pass.

I continue to make baked goods and other treats with nuts and have become comfortable with my chosen lifestyle.

If I stray and fall off my diet one or more of my

symptoms recur. I go back on my diet and they subside.

Conclusion

My quest for wellness has taken me on a long journey. At the time of this writing it has been twenty-eight years since my symptoms first began. For seventeen years I sought help from medical doctors for my ailments and six years after I took personal responsibility for my own health I resolved them on my own. I made a lot of mistakes along the way but I now know what works for me.

Since then I have learned that lifestyle affects the body's ability to heal itself, and alternatives work well for conditions that are self limited or have no known cause.

I'm still insured through an HMO so I sought out and selected an in-network primary care physician who respects the fact that I use natural healing. Even though he is a conventional practitioner I respect him as a professional and I like him as a human being. He uses a teaching approach to healing and is personable, compassionate, and considerate. He listens and takes the time to explain things fully when I ask him a question. I usually leave his office a little more knowledgeable than I was when I went there.

When I need to see him for a diagnosis, I research my options and decide whether or not to fill any prescription he may give me. If a natural remedy has been proven to be as effective I will usually use one. Before deciding to use a natural remedy I make sure I know what I need it for, what it consists of, how safe it is, how effective it is, and how to use it. And I use it responsibly.

If I've been using homeopathic remedies I stop for a couple of days before appointments because homeopathic medicines can alter symptoms and might confuse or astound a conventional practitioner.

When my doctor finds no known cause for an ailment I consult a reference manual, or sometimes a certified herbalist who has a nutritional doctorate and master herbalists degree. (N.D. and M.H.)

For muscular-skeletal ailments (if feasible) I consult my chiropractor for adjustments or acupuncture.

My allergies have increased and I have begun taking allergy shots again. My allergy specialist supports me in my decision to use the paleo diet with the recommendation that I take calcium supplements. I use an herbal calcium supplement that contains magnesium and vitamins

A&D, which are more easily absorbed than calcium carbonate, which is used in most commercial products.

I have become comfortable making decisions that affect my welfare and while it has taken a really long time, I have found a lifestyle that works for me. I continue to research the healing arts and hope to someday overcome my allergies and intolerances, and achieve total wellness.

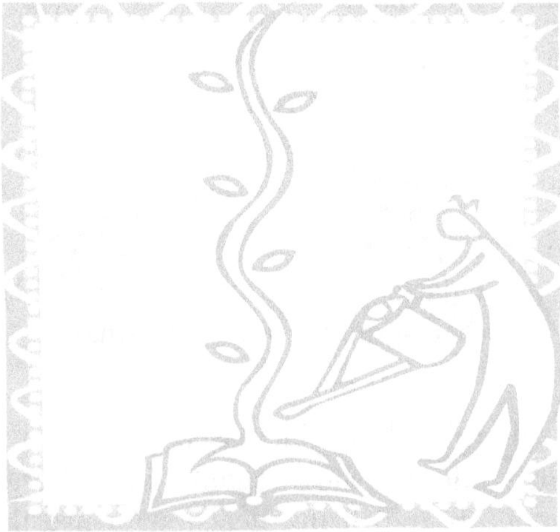

SYMPTOMS

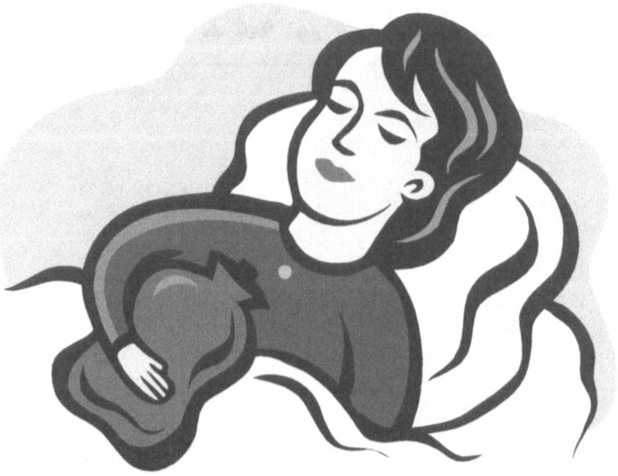

SYMPTOMS

Symptoms are the body's way of telling us when something is wrong.

Conventional medical practitioners look for pathology *(structural or functional changes)* and are taught that approximately eighty-five percent of common ailments have no known cause or are psycho physiological disorders. The drugs they prescribe are designed to counteract symptoms, usually without dealing with the original cause or causes. Symptoms frequently recur, relief is temporary and more symptoms develop.

The use of any medicine natural or synthetic may help temporarily. When symptoms continue to recur it is important to determine the cause. When we choose to control a symptom our body finds another way of getting our attention.

Eczema is a common condition that is often considered to have no known cause. Using hydrocortisone cream or an anti-histamine will suppress the eczema and make it disappear. As soon as the chosen medicine is discontinued the symptom recurs.

If a symptom is suppressed for an extended length of time the body will find another way to make it known that it doesn't like something or there is a problem.

Ear infections or sinus headaches may occur.

If any or all of these symptoms are suppressed and remain suppressed for an extended length of time, later on they may manifest as asthma or emphysema.

When I was experiencing frequent recurring bouts of eczema, ear infections, and sinus headaches, I researched and found information showing that by:

- Keeping a journal and noting my habits I might be able to determine the cause or causes of the aforementioned conditions
- Avoiding any or all of the substances known to cause eczema (p. 129)

I could address the original cause of eczema, ear infection's and sinus headaches resulting in the ability to resolve my symptoms.

Having learned which foods caused which symptoms I have tried to prevent the symptom by using an antihistamine before eating a problem food. One time I took an antihistamine to prevent a headache I knew I would get if I ate popcorn. The antihistamine did its job and I got by without experiencing the typical “popcorn headache” that I would usually get, but the next day I woke up with a severe case of eczema instead.

Now on rare occasions when I plan to have popcorn I wait for the expected headache and then take an antihistamine.

I have found that it is not a good idea to deliberately expose myself to known allergens because it stresses the adrenal system and causes exhaustion, muscle pain, fatigue, and mood swings, resulting in the need for an allergy crisis remedy (p 124). While the remedy is very effective it would not be beneficial to overuse it as that could create problems of its own. The healthiest way to address allergy related symptoms is avoidance of the offending substance or substances whenever possible.

12

TOOLS

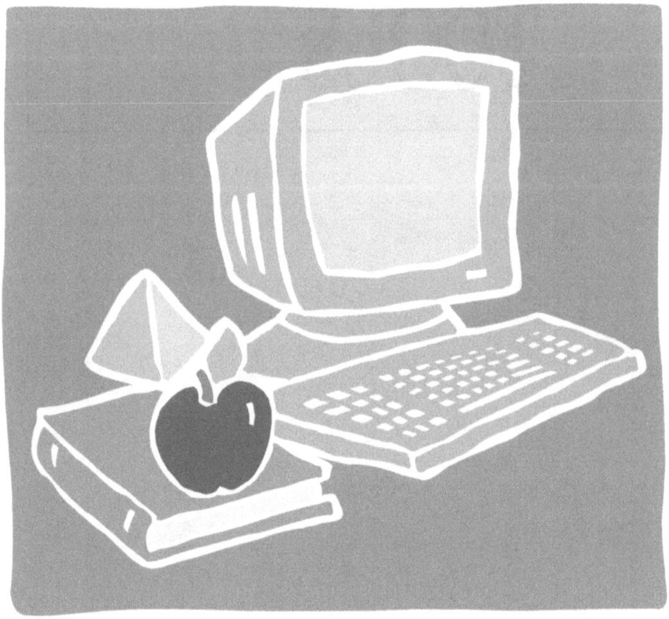

TOOLS

When problems recur or remain unresolved we learn from experience what works and what doesn't. Having the right tools helps us correct our problems more efficiently.

Medical Dictionary- a medical dictionary comes in handy for defining the language used by medical practitioners.

Physicians Desk Reference- a physician's desk reference is helpful for learning about prescription medications, their side effects and contraindications. Even though a doctor has your history, it is a good idea to make sure your prescriptions are right for you.

The Merck Manual of Diagnosis and Therapy- The Merck Manual of Diagnosis and Therapy describes conditions, therapies, and causes, if known. Conditions considered to have no known cause are determined to be psycho physiological disorders. A medical dictionary helped me reference this manual. I found the manual itself preferable over the online or electronic version.

No known cause- Sometimes the doctor says that a condition has no known cause. In that case a good natural healing reference guide is helpful.

Traditional therapies address lifestyle practices and the results those practices produce. Disorders are traced to known physical or stress induced factors and are addressed with time-honored approaches.

Most common ailments are self-limited and resolve themselves on their own in about seven to ten days. If a condition remains unresolved, an underlying cause should be considered as a factor. If there is no known cause, referencing natural health guides or consulting an herbalist with a nutritional doctorate (N.D.) or master herbalists degree (M.H.) may be helpful.

> Natural healing and healthy living support the body in its ability to heal itself. If you are taking prescription drugs then you may benefit from the help of a certified herbalist with an M.H. or N.D.

Before using any substance it is important to learn:

- What the substance is for
- How it works
- How to use it
- Use it responsibly

> It is very important to make sure you understand how to use any substance you plan to put on or into your body.

Over consuming or misusing any substance on a regular basis is abusive and can result in serious consequences. Natural healing methods as well as conventional healing methods have guidelines to ensure correct use.

There are plenty of resources available written by qualified individuals advocating the use of alternatives to conventional medicine. When choosing resources look for reference manuals and handbooks that provide the authors' credentials. Following are some of my favorite reference guides for natural healing.

Prescription For Nutritional Healing by Phyllis A. Balch, CNC and James F Balch, M.D.

A Practical A-to-Z Reference To Drug-Free Remedies using Vitamins, Herbs, and Food Supplements

The Natural Family Doctor: The Comprehensive Self-Help Guide to Health and Natural Medicine – by Andrew Stanway.

A practical comprehensive and authoritative guide to safe natural medicine, and whole health maintenance for the entire family.

Over 1000 natural remedies covering more than 100 ailments. Plan for optimal health at every stage of life.

Prescription for Herbal Healing- An A-Z Reference to Hundreds of Common Disorders and Their Herbal Remedies. by Phyllis A. Balch CNC

Everybody's Guide to Homeopathic Medicines by Stephen Cummings, M.D. and Dana Ullman, M.P.H.

Homeopathic Medicine At Home Natural Remedies For Everyday Ailments And Minor Injuries- By Maesimund B. Panos M.D. and Jane Heimlich

The Family Guide To Homeopathy Symptoms and Natural Solutions By Andrew Lockie

The Women's Guide To Homeopathy by Andrew Lockie, M.D. and Nicola Geddes, M.D. Safe, natural, and effective remedies for fatigue, cystitis, PMS, and other menstrual problems, eating disorders, fertility and pregnancy problems, menopausal symptoms, and other women's ailments.

Optimal Wellness by Ralph Golan M.D.

A-to-Z Self-Care for More Than 100 Common Ailments

Herbs

Herbal medicine is the most ancient form of healthcare in recorded history. Herbs have been used throughout the world for centuries. Extensive scientific documentation exists concerning the use of herbs for most common health problems. Herbs support the body in its ability to heal itself and are processed differently in the body than over the counter medicines or pharmaceutical prescriptions. Herbs enter the body slowly and build up, supporting the body in its ability to heal itself (acute use p58). Because the whole plant is used there are fewer side effects than with synthetic medicines. Herbs are of greatest benefit when we know what we need them for (have a diagnosis), and how to use them. Adverse effects can occur if used improperly.

If you have a recurring symptom that does not respond to herbs there may be an underlying cause that needs to be addressed before healing can occur.

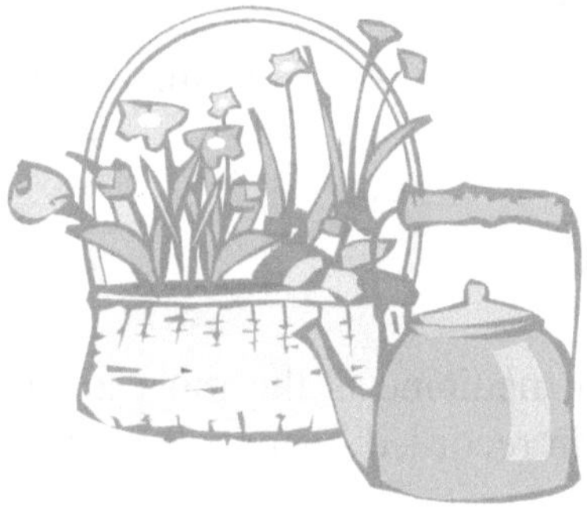

Bach Flower Essences

There are thirty-eight Bach flower essences.

Dr. Edward Bach (1886-1936) noted that emotions affected the body's ability to heal it self and flowers evoked healing.

Dr. Bach researched and selected specific kinds of flowers for healing based on their effects and found a way to extract and preserve the essences derived from them.

Bach Flower Essences are used to reduce stress and other negative emotional states. When the emotional state is eased the physical state is relieved as well, resulting in a more positive outlook and a reduction in stress and stress related disorders. The flower essences are especially helpful following transition, accident, trauma, or grief, and are safe to use with other healing modalities, including conventional medicine.

Rescue Remedy is a combination Bach Flower Essence especially helpful for stress. It is available in different forms. As a tincture that can be administered in a glass of water or directly under the tongue, as an oral spray, as a pill that melts under the tongue, or as a cream that can be rubbed into the pulse points of the neck or wrists. Rescue Remedy Cream can also alleviate muscle tension, spasm, Charlie horse and headaches when rubbed into the affected area.

Homeopathy-homeopathic remedies are symptom specific and efficacious, quickly reducing discomfort and duration time for most self-limited conditions.

It is a healing approach well worth studying. Being familiar with this modality (form of healing) makes remedy selection easy.

Of the more than two thousand remedies available there are twenty-eight commonly used remedies that are practical for home use.

Having a remedy kit and reference book (Tools p90-92) on hand is very helpful for common conditions like diarrhea, flu, poison ivy, sunburn, muscle aches, pains and strains, etc.

My personalized remedy for poison ivy is Rhus Tox, I have used Rusto lotion and Rhus tox to relieve discomfort from poison ivy with immediate results. The itch was gone in minutes and the poison ivy dried up and disappeared within a few days. (There are several remedies for poison ivy, remedy selection should be based on individual symptom's using a homeopathic reference guide)

When one of my dairy goats teats was suddenly red and swollen from mastitis Belladonna 30C eased her condition overnight.

Homeopathics are my preferred healing modality. I have found similarities for the uses of herbs and homeopathics. Chamomile is an herb used for calming, as is homeopathic chamomilla. St. John's Wort is useful for crush injuries and nerve pain as is its homeopathic form Hypericum Perforatum. Being familiar with herbs helps with homeopathic remedy selection.

Acupuncture

Acupuncture is a form of healing based on energy. Energy circulates in the body along twelve major pathways linked to specific internal organs and energy systems. There are over one thousand points along the energy pathways that can be used in acupuncture to direct healing. Acupuncture has been effectively used to treat pain, asthma, bronchitis, migraine, sinus, sciatica, headaches, addictions, hormonal imbalance, menstrual problems, and menopause.

> Through a qualified practitioner there are thousands of conditions for which acupuncture can be used.

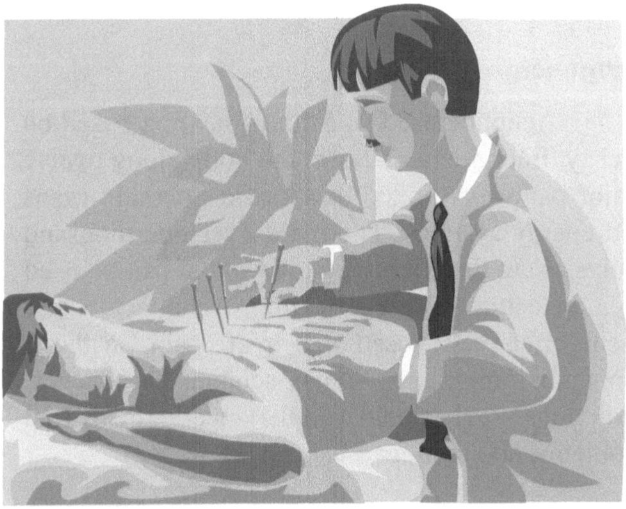

This picture is enlarged to give you an idea about acupuncture, however the actual size of acupuncture needles is much smaller than the ones shown above. The needles my practitioner uses are very tiny and flexible. They are considerably more delicate than the ones depicted here.

CHOICES

Primary Concerns By Sherry Ferrell

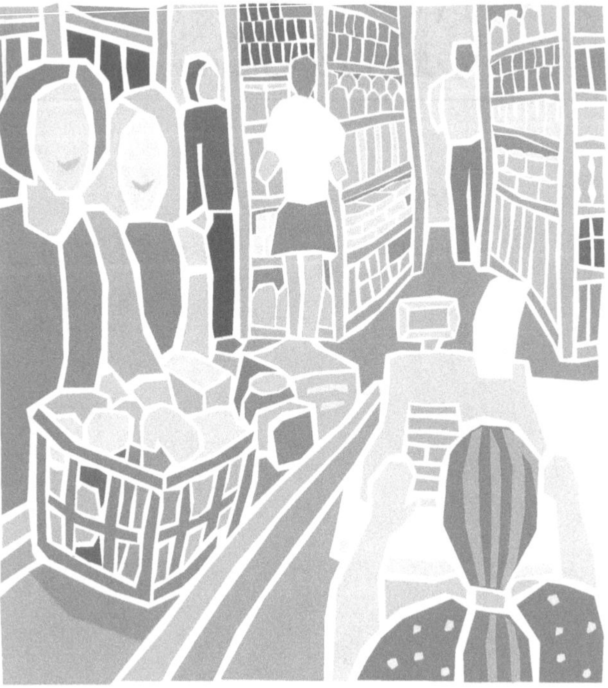

CHOICES

Ideally the healthiest food choices we could make would be one hundred percent natural, totally organic, whole foods. Since organics are not feasible for everyone, choosing foods that are fresh and whole (have not been modified in any way) is far healthier than accepting everyday fare.

The healthy foods our ancestors thrived on have been altered from their natural state (ancient grains have been replaced with hybridized versions that are higher in starch and lower in fiber, and may also contain molds and mycotoxins due to modern storing practices) and replaced with lesser quality ingredients that contribute to poor health.

Lesser quality ingredients are widely available because they are inexpensive and have a longer shelf life than the healthy foods they were derived from.

Foods high in sugars, salt, and the wrong kinds of fat contribute to health problems. Foods made from simple carbohydrates like: processed cereals, doughnuts, muffins, cookies, cakes, candies, sugar, white potatoes, white rice, white bread, and white flour break down very quickly in the digestive system, elevating insulin levels making us tired, creating sugar cravings, and hunger. Many of these foods also contain high fructose corn syrup, and hydrogenated or partially hydrogenated fats, which contribute to coronary artery disease.

Fats

Most commercially available vegetable oils are heat processed and no longer retain their natural nutritional qualities.

Unhealthy Fats like partially hydrogenated and hydrogenated fats are linked to coronary artery disease.

The process of hydrogenation changes the molecular structure of oil, giving it a longer shelf life. Hydrogenated fat is linked to heart attack, stroke, high blood pressure, and arteriosclerosis or hardening of the arteries. Shortening is usually made from hydrogenated fats. Hydrogenated and partially hydrogenated fats are found in many prepackaged foods.

Most convenience foods like coffee creamer, frostings, whipped toppings, bread mixes, cake mixes, cereals, peanut butter, margarines, spreads, shortenings, pizza dough, fried foods, frozen French fries, margarines, and spreads contain unhealthy fats.

When choosing fats look for non-hydrogenated products like Smart Balance non-hydrogenated spread, **expeller pressed**, and **cold pressed** oils, **extra virgin** olive oil, and flaxseed oil.

Salmon oil, flaxseed oil, and walnut oil are high in omega-3 fatty acids. Flaxseed oil is good drizzled on salads and vegetables. Flaxseed oil and cold water fish oils are available in capsule form. Walnut oil is good with vinaigrettes and in baked goods.

Cold pressed and expeller pressed oils have a higher nutritional content than heat processed oils.

Healthy fats help lower cholesterol, provide the body with energy, and stave off hunger. Healthy sources of fats are grass fed organic meats, cold-water fish like salmon and mackerel, nuts and seeds, avocados, olives, and coconuts.

Before the practice of feeding livestock grains instead of pasture grasses to fatten them up quicker, Omega-3 essential fatty acids used to naturally occur in our diets on a two to one ratio with omega-6 essential fatty acids. Changing from grass fed livestock to grain fed livestock changed the omega-3 fats to omega-6 fats increasing the fatty acid ratio to a twenty to one omega-6 to omega-3 fatty acid ratio. *(Loren Cordain, Paleo Diet)*

Increasing our omega-3 consumption through diet and supplementation can ensure we're getting enough omega-3 essential fatty acids.

LIVING FOOD

There are no substitutes for the benefits of a diet that is high in fresh live foods.

Living foods give us energy; provide us with life giving nutrients, and support our body's ability to heal itself.

Vegetables- Raw vegetables are high in fiber and

live enzymes that aid digestion. They provide antioxidants, vitamins, and minerals, and add texture, flavor, color, and variety to our meals.

Include at least one fresh vegetable in each meal every day.

If you have difficulty consuming raw fruits and vegetables add them into your diet slowly or lightly steam them instead of eating them raw. Raw or lightly steamed vegetables like broccoli, carrots, sugar snap peas, peppers, and cauliflower make quick healthy snacks. They are good with salad dressing or dip.

Cauliflower can be mashed like potatoes, *(a handheld stick blender is ideal for creaming cauliflower)* and it goes well with other vegetables like green beans, zucchini, yellow squash, broccoli and carrots. *(Start with small quantities to find out if it gives you gas).* Sweet potatoes and yams are good replacements for white potatoes as well.

Roasted vegetables have a lot of flavor and are easy to prepare. Fresh roasted carrots, onions, yellow squash or zucchini drizzled with olive oil and sprinkled with a little salt and pepper are full of flavor and color.

Roasted chunks of red potatoes with the skins on are fabulous coated with thyme and a little olive oil.

Whole sweet potatoes baked in the oven with the skins on are an excellent accompaniment to a meal and also make a healthy breakfast food, anytime snack, or treat.

If fresh vegetables aren't feasible then frozen are next best, canned as a last resort.

Nuts, Seeds, Fruits and Berries

Raw nuts, seeds, fruits and berries are nature's fast foods. They are high in fiber; provide antioxidants, vitamins and minerals, and live enzymes that aid digestion. They are an excellent replacement for high sugar treats.

Fruits, nuts, seeds, and berries are good nutrient dense foods to start off the day with; they provide lots of energy and also make healthy snacks which lower cholesterol and support heart health.

After being allergy tested and finding out cereals were off limits for me I ate a banana coated in sunflower seeds every morning for breakfast until I figured out what else I could eat. It was a quick satisfying healthy breakfast. Now my daughter and I use raw nuts, seeds, and berries as a replacement for sugar-sweetened cereal.

> Berries are nutrient dense, high in fiber and lower in carbohydrates than other fruits.

I find berries help me curb my cravings for sweets and are especially helpful when I'm trying to lose weight. If fresh berries are not feasible then I use frozen.

Fresh whole fruits containing all their nutritional qualities and fiber are preferable to juices.

> It takes between three and five pieces of fruit to make a large glass of juice, that much juice raises insulin levels and is equivalent to eating candy. It also lacks the fiber and enzymes contained in a piece of fresh fruit.

One of my favorite breakfasts is a small bowl of sliced almonds or chopped pecans topped with fresh or frozen berries and drizzled with just a little bit of honey. Sometimes I add water, almond milk, or apple juice and eat it like cereal (Easy Breakfast p198).

A raw apple with cinnamon, honey and

toasted almond, walnut, or pecan pieces makes a good breakfast. It is also good baked. The texture of the roasted nuts makes up for traditional piecrust.

The monounsaturated fats contained in nuts are very healthy. They provide energy and endurance.

Monounsaturated fats are known to lower blood cholesterol and help prevent artery-clogging arteriosclerosis.

The healthy fats in nuts are an excellent energy source. I find nuts satisfy me longer than other snacks.

Grinding nuts and seeds makes them more digestible.

Nuts that have been ground can replace flour in bread recipes.

I buy raw nuts at a wholesale buying club and store them in the refrigerator or freezer if they are not going to be used right away.

- **Almonds-** sometimes referred to as the king of nuts are related to peaches. They are rich in protein, phosphorus, magnesium, calcium, vitamin E, monounsaturated fats, omega-6 essential fatty acids, and are high in fiber. One ounce of almonds contains six grams of carbohydrate and three grams of fiber, which reduces the total carbohydrate count to three grams per ounce. A one-ounce serving of nuts can curb hunger for two to four hours.

Raw almonds can be sprouted to increase the already exceptional nutritional content.

Almonds can be used for making breads, as a replacement for cereal and for making cookies, cakes, pie crusts, almond milk, custards, frozen desserts, and roasted almond butter; a healthier alternative to peanut butter *(which contains molds known as aflatoxins, that are suspected carcinogens*).

Roasted almond butter is good spread on a banana, on fresh slices of apple, or on celery sticks. Sometimes we make almond butter and *low-sugar jelly sandwiches on nut flour bread. It is especially good on almond-pecan flour bread (low sugar jelly p201).

- **Brazil nuts** are high in selenium, and combine well with almond flour for baking, however, because of the higher fat content in brazil nuts; eliminating or reducing the amount of oil in recipes is recommended.

- **Cashews**- belonging to the sumac family of plants are nutrient rich and high in carbohydrates. They are good roasted for snacks and for making roasted cashew butter, which can be used as a spread. (I like it spread on an apple slice)

- **Hazelnuts or filberts-** are nutrient rich and contain monounsaturated fats. They are fragrant and flavorful and blend well with almond flour for baking.

- **Pecans**-are related to the hickory family of nuts, are nutrient rich and high in essential fatty acids. Pecans combine well with almonds for making nut flour for baking bread.

- **Pumpkin seeds** are rich in protein, iron,

and phosphorus, and contain calcium, niacin, and zinc. They are good eaten as snacks or combined with dried fruits, sprinkled on fresh fruits or on salads. Pumpkin and squash seeds can be eaten raw, dried, shelled, and roasted.

- Raw **sesame seeds-**are very high in calcium; and are a healthy satisfying treat. So is sesame butter or tahini_(ta-hee-nee). It can be used as a dip or spread. Tahini can be found in the international food section of some grocery stores.

- **Sunflower seeds** are rich in vitamin E, and are very high in calcium. They are good as snacks or sprinkled on salads.

- **Walnuts**- contain omega-3 essential fatty acids, are good added to salads, baked goods, whole grains, cereals, and sprinkled on desserts and snacks. Walnuts have a higher starch content than other nuts; and when made into flour for baking, lend a pleasant sponge like texture to the finished product.

If you are trying to lose weight use fruit, nuts, and honey, in moderation. A serving size of nuts is one quarter of a cup.

Water

One of the healthiest things we can do for ourselves is to drink plenty of clean pure water. It transports nutrients through the body and is essential for removing waste. On average we need a minimum of eight eight-ounce glasses of water each and every day, more if we are overweight.

Other beverages like fruit juice, coffee, tea, or soda, are processed in the body differently and do not make up for drinking water. Many of these beverages contain the wrong kinds of sweeteners or caffeine that cause fluctuations in our energy levels and cravings.

> The regular consumption of drinks containing aspartame and splenda can lead to symptoms of chronic fatigue, fibromyalgia, and symptoms similar to multiple sclerosis (MS). Medical doctors have not yet attributed a cause for these baffling symptoms. Sufferers who have stopped using splenda and aspartame have obtained relief.

Beverages that contain high fructose corn syrup contribute to poor health (p115). Creamers used in coffee and tea contain hydrogenated fat (p100).

Drinking plenty of pure clean water to satisfy thirst will support the body's ability to cleanse itself.

Constipation, boils and blemishes, sinus congestion, and lingering cough are just a few symptoms of not drinking enough water. Once anything is added to water the chemical composition changes and it is not water anymore. **There is no substitute for pure water.**

One of the best ways to insure the quality of your drinking water would be to invest in a filtration system. (I did a lot of research on water filtration systems before making an investment and my personal preference for insuring the integrity of my drinking water is the British Berkefield filtering system. The British Berkefield filtering system is available online).

Milk

Fresh non-pasteurized milk is a living food that contains enzymes, which support digestion. The heat process used to pasteurize (kill bacteria) milk destroys the enzymes.

Research shows that milk is high in hidden sugar, is difficult to digest and causes excess mucus in the body. Dairy products are linked to conditions such as ear infections, chronic runny nose, post-nasal drip, cough, sinusitis, allergies, and asthma.

After experiencing frequent ear infections, congestion, post-nasal drip, eczema and irritable bowel syndrome I learned that milk was not a healthy food for me. When I began to research the aforementioned conditions I found a common factor in all of them. That factor appeared to be, the consumption of dairy products.

If you tolerate dairy products well, the best choices are **kefir**, and **yogurt** as they are easier to digest.

The healthiest brands contain **live active cultures** of beneficial bacteria that promote digestive health.

Look for organic and hormone free yogurts and kefir.

Some yogurts contain added starch for thickening, high fructose corn syrup, or artificial sweeteners that can contribute to poor health. Read labels.

Plain yogurt sweetened with a little honey and vanilla, topped with fresh fruit, and sprinkled with some toasted walnuts, almonds, or pecans, makes a satisfying healthy treat.

Meat

Fresh lean meats like: chicken, fish, pork, and beef provide complete proteins that help oxygenate red blood cells and build muscle mass for strength and endurance. By combining incomplete proteins a complete protein can be made but the results are different in that oxygenation levels drop and muscle mass reduces.

Processed meats like: cold cuts, hot dogs, bacon, sausage, and fried chicken, can contain hidden sugars, salt, or hydrogenated fats, contributing to sugar imbalance, high blood pressure, and coronary artery disease.

Health food stores have better alternatives to processed meats but the cost is considerably higher.

A quick healthy sausage patty can be easily made from fresh ground pork by adding dry ingredients like sage, or dried ground peppers and just a little salt (p202*)*.

Organic Grass fed meats are optimum containing healthy omega-3 fats. They are however usually more expensive than commercial meat products. If grass-fed meats are not feasible then supplementing with omega-3 fish oil or flaxseed oil will help balance the omega-6 to omega-3 fatty acid ratio. Grass fed organic meats are now available in some upscale grocery stores.

Sweeteners

Any sweetener used in excess can contribute to poor health. If you are concerned about high cholesterol, overweight, or insulin related disorders, curbing conventional sweets can help considerably. The kinds of sweeteners used in everyday fare can raise triglyceride levels and contribute to increased cholesterol, especially high fructose corn syrup, which is 42-90 percent fructose. Most fructose available as a sweetener is derived from corn as opposed to the healthy fructose that occurs naturally in fruit.

Honey is a simple sugar, which is twice as sweet as table sugar but more easily digested. Using honey in place of granulated sugar reduces sugar cravings and helps lower cholesterol. Honey like any sugar should be used sparingly. *Honey should not be given to children under two years of age because their digestive tracts and immune systems are not yet developed enough for bacteria that may be present in honey.*

Sugar- is known to cause fluctuations in insulin levels causing cravings, creating a vicious cycle of more cravings for sugar.

Sugar is linked to known conditions such as hypoglycemia, diabetes, and Polycystic Ovarian Syndrome.

Cane sugar, sugar cane, cane juice, brown sugar, sucanot, and molasses are all sugar products.

High fructose corn syrup is widely available because it costs less to produce than other sweeteners like granulated sugar. It is contained in many of the foods we eat every day and is known to cause poor health. It can be found in most prepared and prepackaged foods including beverages.

High fructose corn syrup is converted from corn syrup and contains 42% - 90% fructose.

Studies have shown that it raises triglyceride levels and increases the risk of coronary artery disease.

Artificial sweeteners- may hinder weight loss and contribute to poor health. Artificial sweeteners can be difficult to digest. If you have poor digestive health or any inflammation in your body you may want to avoid sweeteners other than honey. Canker sores are an indication of inflammation in the digestive system. Using Splenda, Stevia, and products containing fructooligosaccharides can cause canker sores in some people.

Aspartame and splenda have been linked to chronic fatigue, fibromyalgia, headaches, muscle stiffness, joint pain and symptoms similar to multiple sclerosis.

Stevia- is considered a healthy alternative to sugar. Stevia is sold in the nutritional supplements section of health food stores. Our government does not allow it to be sold as a sweetener. If you have any digestive health problems you may want to avoid stevia.

Date Sugar-comes from dried dates and is available through health food stores and food co-ops. Date sugar can be used cup for cup as a replacement for granulated sugar in baked goods. Reduce oven temperature twenty-five degrees.

Making date sugar is easy with a food processor. Just pulse until the dates are finely ground and you're done. Dates are high in starch.

Fruit juice concentrate- a concentrated source of natural sugar that lacks fiber and can cause rapid fluctuations in blood sugar levels.

Fructose - is a natural sugar found in fruits and plants. Common commercially available fructose is derived from cornstarch. Fructose is linked to increased LDL cholesterol levels, uric-acid levels, and elevated triglyceride levels.

Maple Syrup- is a concentrated sweetener, which can cause rapid fluctuations in blood sugar levels. If used in excess can offset the acid alkaline balance.

Brown Rice Syrup – available at health food stores and co-ops. Rice syrup is digested slowly reducing fluctuations in blood sugar levels.

Salt

Salt should be used sparingly or avoided if you have high blood pressure. Sea salt and brown salt (Real Salt), which contain natural minerals, are healthy alternatives to commercial varieties. Look for sodium on food labels.

Flour

- **Whole grain wheat flour** is a

living food, which contains nutritional oils that support and build the body. It is also high in fiber, which is good for healthy digestion and elimination. The grain can be stored for weeks or months and will retain its nutrients until it is ground for making flour. Grains that are kept too long will develop a rancid smell and flavor.

- **Bleached or enriched white flour** is derived from whole-wheat berries (grains). The healthy oils and fiber are removed to increase the shelf life and give it a lighter or fluffier texture than whole grain wheat flour.

Because white flour lacks fiber it is high in carbohydrates and quickly turns to sugar during digestion. Lack of fiber slows digestion and elimination.

The process used to produce enriched white flour removes all of the health giving properties making the flour completely devoid of nutrients. It can be called enriched simply by adding a few chemical nutrients back in.

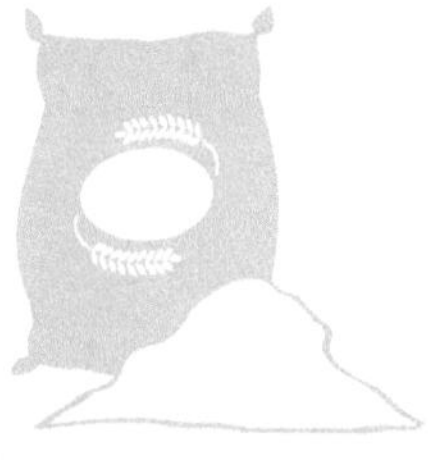

COMMON AILMENTS

Primary Concerns By Sherry Ferrell

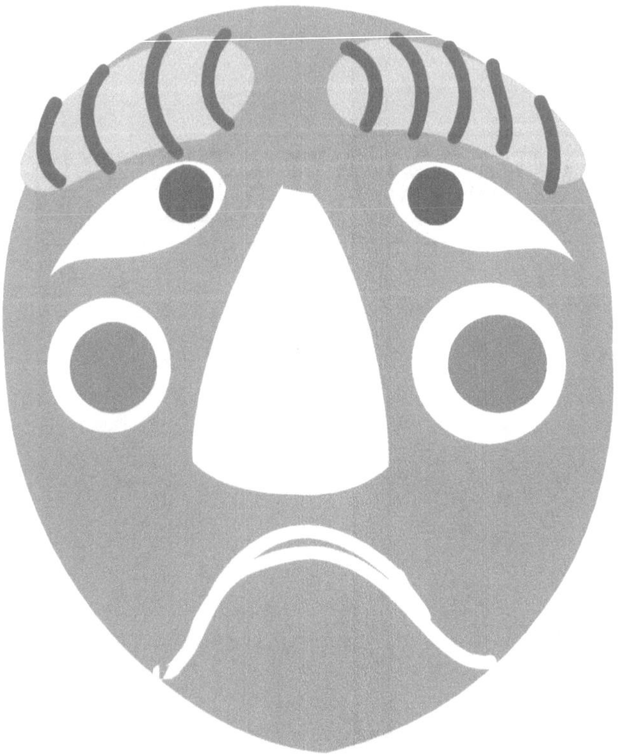

COMMON AILMENTS

Acid Reflux

> Too much stomach acid may not always be the cause of heartburn, or acid reflux. A lack of digestive enzymes presents with symptoms that are very similar.

A simple way to find out if you have too much stomach acid or not enough stomach acid is to eat a pickle or take a tablespoon of vinegar, fresh lemon juice, or pickle juice. If you experience an increase in symptoms, there is too much acid. If your symptoms improve then there is not enough acid to digest your food. Supplementing with digestive enzymes and consuming more raw fruits and vegetables can help increase enzyme production.

Ideally enzymes come from a healthy diet of fresh living foods.

If you have difficulty consuming raw fruits and vegetables add them into your diet slowly or lightly steam them instead of eating them raw, then gradually increase the raw amount. Because the heat process during cooking destroys enzymes it is important to include a raw food at every meal or snack.

Cultured foods also help to improve digestion by balancing the intestinal flora. Look for cultured products such as **miso**, pronounced me-so (a fermented soup base found at health food stores) **sauerkraut** *(Check the deli section of the market for quality sauerkraut),* **kefir** *(more liquid than yogurt, contains higher number of cultured bacteria),* or **yogurt**. <u>Check labels for live active cultures.</u> Commercial yogurts that contain starches, high fructose corn syrup, or artificial sweeteners contribute to poor health.

Lemons-Squeezing a fresh lemon first thing every morning, adding the juice to an eight-ounce glass of water, and sipping the contents can help improve digestion and help to tone and regulate the bowels.

Enzyme supplements can help to improve digestion and are usually available at herb shops and health food stores.

Allergies and intolerances can affect the body in different ways. Gastroenteropathy, inflammation, swelling, rashes, headaches, muscle and joint pain, fatigue, anxiety, and increased pulse are just a few indications of allergic reactions or intolerances.

Repeated exposure to substances that cause allergic reactions or intolerances however mild can lead to chronic muscle pain and stiffness, chronic rhinitis, chronic sinus, and physical exhaustion.

Most conventional practitioners have been taught that food allergy and intolerance are predominantly psycho physiologic conditions.

Unlike an allergy, intolerance does not initiate an antibody reaction so testing does not always indicate known or unknown causes for food related problems.

Severe allergic reactions can cause rapid heartbeat, difficulty breathing, or shock, and in some cases may even be fatal.

Repeated upper respiratory infections, ear infections, congestion, runny nose, cough, and sinusitis may indicate allergies or intolerances as underlying causes.

Reactive hypoglycemia is a condition that is often seen in conjunction with allergies and intolerances.

If you suspect you may have allergies or intolerances a simple pulse test might prove helpful in making a determination.

Check your resting heart rate before meals and again thirty minutes after meals. If your resting heart rate increases by a count of fifteen or more you may have food allergies or intolerances.

Repeated exposure to substances that one is allergic or intolerant to can stress the adrenal system causing low body temperature, fatigue, nervousness, tension, or weakened immunity to infections, resulting in an allergy crisis. An herbal allergy formula can help restore balance during an allergy crisis. My personal preference is 500mg DGL licorice root, 200mg ginseng extract in capsules, and 250mg pantothenic acid. It is important to determine the source of allergens and avoid them if possible.

Sometimes making a determination on your own can be difficult.

Allergy and intolerance can affect any area of the body.

The help of a highly qualified allergy specialist is recommended. It is my experience that test results can vary depending on who does the testing. Ask friends and acquaintances who they would recommend.

Arthritis- is an inflammatory condition that responds well to the elimination of beans, grains, dairy products, sugars, and sweeteners other than honey. Try curbing these foods for two to three weeks and see if there is a reduction in symptoms. (see paleo diet p148)

The consumption of beverages other than water, especially sodas, can contribute to muscle pain, stiffness, and joint pain, which are indicators of toxic overload. When the liver is overloaded its ability to remove impurities from the body can become impaired and inflammation may result. Eliminating soda from your diet and drinking water can reduce or resolve discomfort attributed to toxic overload. Drinking plenty of pure fresh water allows the body to cleanse itself, reducing inflammation, stiffness and pain.
For more information on the benefits of drinking clean pure water see pages 110-111.

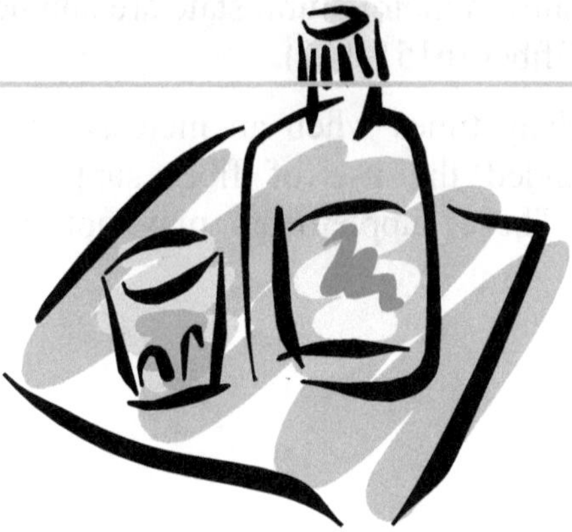

Constipation

Some common reasons for constipation are not drinking enough water, not consuming enough fresh fruits and vegetables, and the use of certain prescription medications.

Nuts, seeds, berries, and fresh fruits and vegetables are high in fiber and regular consumption helps to regulate the bowels (also see lemons p122).

If you suddenly increase the fiber content of your diet too much you may experience some discomfort because your body needs time to adjust to a change from the amount of fiber it normally receives. If you are not used to consuming fresh foods a sudden increase can cause diarrhea. To avoid this problem slowly increase your consumption of fresh fruits and vegetables or lightly steam them and slowly increase the amount until they become a regular part of your diet.

If you have a healthy digestive system whole grains in their natural state are another good source of fiber (p151-167).

Many times when an increase in fiber is recommended the use of fiber supplements is advised. These supplements may not work for everyone.

In some people fiber supplements have the opposite effect and can increase constipation instead of resolving it.

Constipation is another condition that is often considered to be a psycho physiological disorder by some physicians.

IRRITIBLE BOWEL SYNDROME

By a ratio of three to one women are more commonly affected by irritable bowel syndrome than men and the cause is considered to be stress related. Anti-spasmotics and anti-depressants are usually prescribed. A normal diet is recommended. If spastic colon or constipation is present an increase in dietary fiber is advised.

Common illnesses that may be confused with IBS are lactose intolerance and allergic gastroenteropathy. *(Merck Manual of Diagnosis and Therapy)*

> Current information is available that shows a correlation between irritable bowel syndrome, inflammation of the digestive system, and the consumption of sugars and starches (p145).

Recurring headaches can be an indication of food intolerance or other underlying disorders. Sinus headaches can be caused by sensitivities to foods and also by environmental sensitivities such as mold, pollen, and animal dander. If left untreated sinus infections can occur.

I experienced frequent headaches and recurring ear infections for many years before I realized they were caused by allergies to foods (corn, rice, and rye) and sensitivities to grass pollens. Eventually I realized antihistamines alleviated headaches that did not respond to analgesics. Discovering and eliminating what I was sensitive to alleviated my symptoms. Eliminating grains from my diet helped alleviate symptoms associated with environmental sensitivities to grass pollen (p 65).

For stress induced headaches rescue remedy and other Bach Flower Essences can be helpful.

The regular use of analgesics can become addictive.

I once had a co-worker who experienced regular headaches as withdrawal symptoms from the recurrent use of analgesics. She found that it took two to three weeks of avoidance to correct the problem.

Eczema is a common condition sometimes considered to have no known cause. The itching from this condition can be much worse than the itch associated with poison ivy.

When I was suffering with recurring bouts of eczema I went to my family doctor, was diagnosed with dermatitis and prescribed cortisone cream to suppress the symptoms. I used the recommended treatment for many years for relief from that condition but it recurred frequently.

Through researching alternative resources I learned that eczema is considered to be an outward sign of an inner problem. If suppressed for an extended length of time eczema can manifest as a more serious condition such as asthma or emphysema.

Lack of digestive enzymes, intestinal inflammation, and food allergies and intolerances are known to produce eczema in some people. Some of the foods commonly known to cause eczema are; chocolate, citrus, dairy, eggs, peanuts, corn and wheat.

My doctor says he sees a lot of eczema in winter. In winter we lose moisture due to the drying effects of our heating systems. The use of a humidifier can help decrease the risk of excessively dry skin. Sponge bathing two or three days out of the week instead of taking tub baths or showers can help keep skin hydrated.

Using moisturizer or skin cream can help with dry skin. Read labels and avoid chemicals, especially aluminum that is linked to Alzheimer's. Healthy skin care products are available through health food stores and herb shops.

Ear infections

Recurring ear infections can be an indication of an underlying disorder such as allergies or intolerances to foods or other substances such as mold, pollen, chemicals, or animal dander. Dairy products are linked to conditions such as, ear infections, chronic runny nose, post-nasal drip, cough, sinusitis, allergies, and asthma. Ear infections can resolve themselves as long as the offending substance is avoided.

If a course of antibiotics (natural or prescription) is used replacing intestinal flora *(following treatment)* with a probiotic is recommended. Probiotics are available at herb shops, health food stores, and at some pharmacies, and grocery stores.

Chronic Fatigue and Fibromyalgia

Chronic fatigue and fibromyalgia are often experienced in conjunction with one another.

Chronic fatigue is another condition often considered to have no known cause or as being a psycho physiological condition. Chronic fatigue is not entirely understood by conventional medical practitioners.

Improper diet, environmental sensitivities, food allergies and intolerances, too much sugar, lack of sufficient rest, refined foods; fast foods, excess caffeine or alcohol may cause chronic fatigue in some people.

Chronic fatigue, fibromyalgia, and MS like symptoms have been linked to the regular consumption of sodas and other beverages containing splenda, or aspartame.

I experienced chronic fatigue and fibromyalgia following treatment for injuries sustained in an automobile accident. I later found that chronic fatigue and fibromyalgia are often experienced after an accident or trauma.

Fibromyalgia is a painful condition that often affects those who suffer from chronic fatigue. Fibromyalgia consists of muscle pain, and or tenderness of joint tendons and surrounding soft tissues. Any of the fibro muscular tissues can be involved. Fibromyalgia is often found in conjunction with food allergies and intolerances. Ibs (p131) is another condition often seen in conjunction with chronic fatigue and fibromyalgia.

Canker sores are another common disorder considered to have no known cause, but several factors point toward a localized immune reaction. Canker sores may occur singly or in groups and frequently recur lasting for approximately ten days to two weeks. The acute painful phase lasts for approximately three or four days. Symptoms then diminish spontaneously. Women are affected more often than men. Stress and local trauma are considered to be the predominant precipitating factors related to the cause of canker sores. Treatment may consist of topical anesthetics, oral mouth rinses containing tetracycline, or corticosteroid therapy. *(Merck Manual of Diagnosis and Therapy)*

(Deficiencies of iron, B-12, and folic acid increase susceptibility). (before supplementing with iron it is important to be sure through laboratory testing that there is an actual deficiency; because too much iron through supplementation can be really bad for you and very difficult to recover from). If iron supplementation is required an herbal formula might be preferable to a chemical formula, which commonly causes constipation as a side effect. Look for iron supplements at herb stores or health food stores. Herbal iron supplements are available in liquid or capsule form).

In some people canker sores are related to food intolerance and disappear after the offending foods are removed from the diet.

Some foods that may cause canker sores in

sensitive individuals are beef, walnuts, beans, cinnamon gum, Splenda, stevia, and fructooligosaccharides.

Temporomandibular Joint Syndrome

Temporomandibular Joint Syndrome or TMJ is defined as pain and inflammation in the joint (the joint on either side of the jaw that opens and closes the mouth) temples and the adjoining muscles, including the back of the head and the neck. It predominantly affects women and is considered to be a stress related disorder. Anti-depressants and sometimes tranquilizers are the recommended treatment.

After enduring several frequent recurring conditions for many years I developed chronic pain in my jaw, the base of my head, neck, and temples.

After discontinuing the use of non-steroidal anti-inflammatory drugs and anti-depressants, being tested for allergies and food intolerance, and then removing foods I was allergic or intolerant to from my diet, the TMJ disappeared.

Rubbing Rescue Remedy cream into the affected areas can help alleviate symptoms.

Menopause While menopause is not an ailment it is a common concern for many women.

The signs of approaching menopause known as peri-menopause may begin as early as age thirty and last for ten years or more. Some women breeze through the peri-menopausal years with hardly any symptoms while others may experience all of them. Some of the signs of approaching menopause may include fatigue, irritability, hot flashes, night sweats, chills, insomnia, headaches, sensations of something crawling on the skin, stress and anxiety.

Traditional approaches to menopause support the body during this transition.

Stress and anxiety are common side effects that may be eased by the use of Bach flower essences. **The Bach Flower Essence** (p93) **Walnut** is especially helpful for stress related to change.

Calcium supplementation is recommended to maintain bone health and cardiovascular system support. Supplements should include magnesium and vitamin D for absorption. Calcium citrate and herbal calcium combinations are more easily assimilated in the body than chemical formulas.

Some herbal formulas for menopause may contain soy and black cohosh, which may not agree with everyone. If you are sensitive to some of the ingredients used in combination formulas for menopause you may benefit from the assistance of a Master Herbalist (M.H.), or certified herbalist with a Nutritional Doctorate (N.D.).

Having had problems with black cohosh and soy I've found 500 mgs of DGL licorice root and a large mug of dandelion root, chamomile, and red raspberry leaf tea first thing every morning to be very helpful. I place one of each tea bag in a four cup glass measuring cup, add boiling water and let steep 3-5 minutes. This makes four servings, which can be saved in the refrigerator for reheating later or enjoyed as iced tea.

Nutritional supplements used for menopause include vitamins A, C E, and calcium. *(Vitamin E can contribute to heavy menstrual flow*).

A diet high in fresh fruits and vegetables can help support the body during this transition and may reduce symptoms.

The use of hormone replacement therapy

through conventional medicine has been linked to serious health risks and side effects in some women.

Some of the "natural" formula's through prescription may be synthetic.

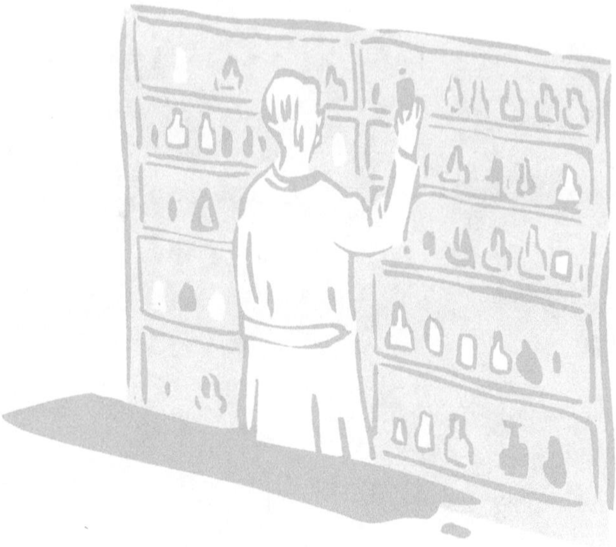

GLUTEN INTOLERANCE

GLUTEN INTOLERANCE

Gluten intolerance is a serious condition that can be fatal if left untreated.

Gluten is a protein found in certain kinds of grains belonging to the wheat family of plants. Wheat, barley, rye, oats, spelt, teff, and kamut are gluten-containing grains. In sensitive individuals gluten can cause inflammation in the digestive tract. Over time the villi, pronounced vil-i *(the villi rise above the mucus that coats the lining of the small intestine and absorb nutrients and fluids)* in the small intestine can begin to break down and erode.

Gluten intolerance is commonly misdiagnosed and can be mistaken for less serious conditions. Sufferers are frequently passed off as being neurotic and given anti-depressants, or more commonly diagnosed as having irritable bowel syndrome, which has no known cause and shows no obvious abnormalities.

Many times a patient with gluten sensitivity or intolerance can unknowingly have the condition for years then during the latent stages when a lot of damage to the lining of the small intestines has already occurred, they may finally be diagnosed. Usually by then there is obvious malabsorption of nutrients and sometimes-irreversible damage to the villi that promote digestion. In severe cases an inability to derive nutrients from food may result. If left undetected damage to the digestive system can become permanent and sometimes fatal. Risk factors for certain forms of cancer are increased for gluten intolerant individuals.

Better testing methods for gluten sensitivity are currently being devised.

In the United States the number of persons per population having gluten sensitivity may be as high as one in two hundred and fifty.

Because gluten intolerance often affects families it is important to test immediate family members of sensitive individuals.

DIETS

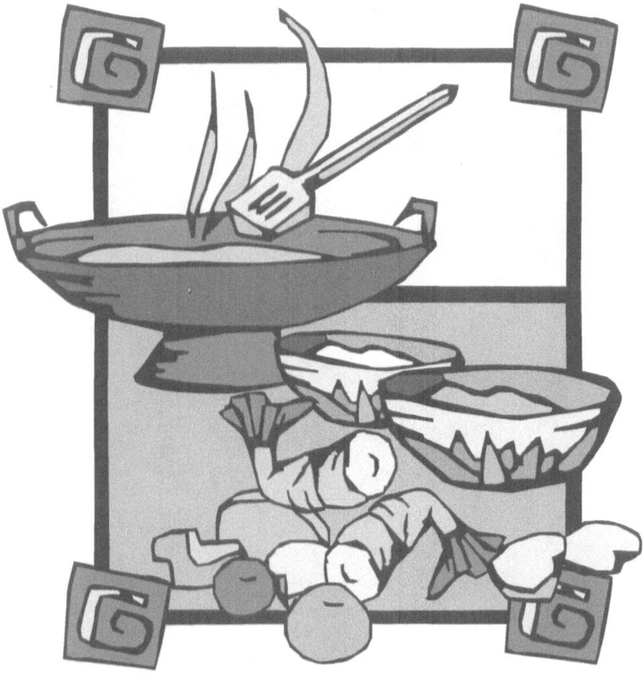

DIETS

One of the first things I noticed when I began studying natural healing and healthy living was that a great deal of emphasis was placed on whole grains. I have since learned from personal experience that grains may not necessarily be healthy for everyone.

For many years I had lived with unexplained hunger that could not be satisfied and physical discomfort related to my diet. At that time I hadn't noticed the connection as an inability to digest sugars and starches.

After trying the Atkins diet and going completely off grains, sugars and starches, and then adding them back in to my diet I noticed I had ravenous hunger ten to twenty minutes after eating, abdominal discomfort and excess gas. I had lived with those symptoms all of my life and had accepted them as normal. When I was avoiding sugars and starches all of the symptoms had disappeared. The symptoms reappeared when I was eating sugars and starches again.

When it became obvious to me that I had problems digesting sugars and starches I began to seek out information regarding that discovery.

Through research documented information became available showing a relationship between inflammation of the digestive system and sugars and starches and I drew my own conclusions.

I noticed problems not only with natural sugars but artificial sweeteners as well. And later found information that coincided with my own experiences.

I had already found I was intolerant to grains and dairy products and eliminating them from my diet brought about a cessation of inflammatory conditions such as eczema, muscle and joint pain, and edema. Lower back pain and Irritable Bowel Syndrome were noticeably improved as well.

Now with the realization that sugars and starches were involved, and by applying what had been revealed to me I was on my way to living symptom free for the first time in my life.

When doing research on the Internet I found many websites with advice concerning diet and IBS, but not all of them provided information that was practical for me.

The following websites, when I applied the information they revealed to me concerning my health, were most beneficial.

- www.healingcrow.com
- www.scdiet.org
- www.paleofood.com

Breaking The Vicious Cycle *Intestinal Health Through Diet* By Elaine Gottschall B.A.,M. Sc. was being promoted on the scdiet.org website. I bought the book, which I found easy to read. The book includes recipes that I decided to tweak to suit my personal preferences. Today, the SCD is being used successfully by many to treat the following: Autism, Crohn's disease, Ulcerative Colitis, Celiac disease, Cystic Fibrosis, Chronic Diarrhea, Candidiasis, and Irritable Bowel Syndrome (IBS). (Excerpted from the healing crow website, specific carbohydrate diet page @ http://www.healingcrow.com/dietsmain/scd/scd.html)

Support and recipes for the specific carbohydrate diet are available on the internet at www.scdiet.org.

Additional Specific Carbohydrate Diet recipes can also be found at www.scdrecipe.com and pecanbread.com a website for those with autism.

Many of the baked goods recipes from the specific carbohydrate diet are made with almond flour. The use of lactose free dairy products is allowed.

I tried the diet for several weeks; hoping the elimination of lactose would make a difference, but my ears started ringing and I experienced an increase in eczema.

Even though this diet turned out to be less than ideal for me, I learned that some of my problems with foods stem from my inability to digest disaccharides *(containing two sugar molecules),* and polysaccharides *(contain two or more sugar molecules, i.e. complex sugar or starch)* and which foods fall into those categories.

I returned to the website www.healingcrow.com and learned about the paleo diet. Most of the techniques I learned from the specific carbohydrate diet applied to the paleo diet. I'm glad I had read Elaine Gottschall's book before I tried the Paleo diet because when I had some adverse reactions to arrowroot, chestnuts, walnuts, and dates I was able to determine the cause. Research showed that the starch content of these foods is high.

It has been approximately five years since I started the paleo diet, which is grain-free, bean-free, potato-free, dairy-free and sugar-free.

INGREDIENTS USED ARE: meat, fish, poultry, vegetables, fruits, nuts, seeds, berries and honey. Fats from meats, olives, and coconuts are used. Paleo Diet recipes on the Internet can be seen at www.paleofood.com. The website has an extensive collection of recipes.

I like perusing www.paleodiet.com which has links to many websites with articles and information on topics concerning the Paleo or Stone-Age Diet.

Being allergic to dairy products, mustard, kale, and broccoli, I take calcium supplements to ensure adequate calcium intake.

Having an issue with weight I was relieved to learn that intentional weight gain, or loss on the aforementioned diet can be controlled through increased or decreased consumption of nuts, honey, and fruits. *(Weight gain may be achieved by increasing consumption of nuts, fruits, and honey. To lose weight, reduce consumption of nuts, fruit, and honey).*

GRAINS

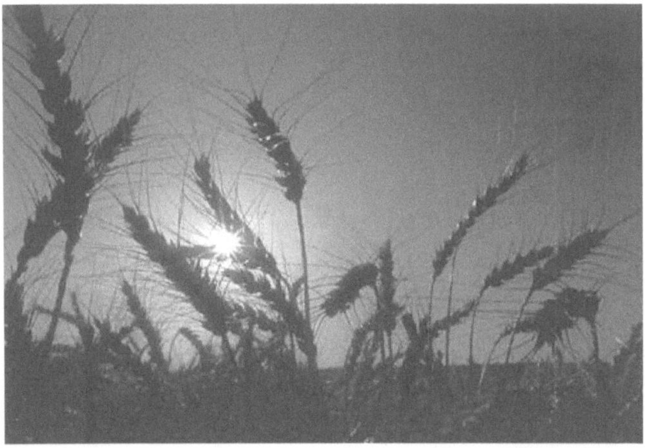

GRAINS

> This book is about transitions and making changes to suit personal needs. This section is for those who tolerate grains well. If you are sensitive to mold, have any kind of inflammation *(ibs, fibromyalgia, arthritis, etc.),* or insulin related conditions (diabetes, polycystic ovarian syndrome, etc.), you may want to curb your consumption of grains, especially wheat and corn (primarily because these grains can harbor mold because of the way they are stored and also because they have been modified)

Before I realized grains were off limits for me I learned a lot about their benefits and uses. I milled organic whole grain flours for making fresh healthy breads and pastas and ground my own cooking cereals.

Many different grains are available through food co-ops and health food stores, allowing for greater variety and nutrients. Unrefined whole grains contain healthy oils, fiber, and nutrients that are lost during the refining process.

Because wheat is such a common ingredient in our food supply I have listed it first.

The best place to store grains is the refrigerator or in a cool place at temperatures less than sixty-five degrees.

Freezing grains overnight in the deep freeze before storing them at room temperature can prevent them from "hatching bugs". Just be sure they are dry before sealing them in an airtight container.

- **Wheat-** is the grain **white all-purpose flour** is derived from. The refining process involves removing the fiber (bran) and the kernel (germ) containing the oils and nutrients to lighten the product (make it fluffy) and extend the shelf life. Some of the nutrients are added back in and it is called enriched white flour.

- **One hundred percent whole grain wheat** is a whole food that contains healthy fiber, oils, and nutrients.

The easiest way to change from a diet containing white flour to a diet containing one hundred percent whole-grain wheat flour is to make small changes gradually. If you increase the fiber content of your diet too much you may experience some discomfort because your body needs time to adjust to a change in the amount of fiber it normally receives.

One way to become accustomed to eating whole-wheat is to buy a loaf of one hundred percent whole wheat bread or a box of one hundred percent whole-wheat cereal or crackers, sampling a very small portion every day. Start slow and increase the portion size gradually.

If you buy a loaf of one hundred percent whole-grain wheat bread and you are the only person in your house eating it you may want to extend the shelf life.

To extend the shelf life of a loaf of bread you can put the slices you won't be eating right away in sandwich bags and insert them back into the original wrapper then freezing them. Later you can take the portions of bread out of the freezer without having to separate them.

When taking the bread from the freezer remove the slices from the sandwich bag before thawing to prevent them from being soggy.

Labels can be misleading so be selective and check the ingredients listed on the package. It should state one hundred percent whole grain wheat. Some manufacturers color the bread to hide the fact that it is mostly all purpose white flour.

Because cereal and crackers have a longer shelf life freezing them is not necessary.

If you would like to try baking with whole-wheat flour a good way to get started is by buying a bag of whole-wheat flour and freezing most of it *(to retain the integrity of the oils)* saving some out for immediate use. When you are baking you can replace a small amount of the white flour you would normally use in your recipe with whole-wheat flour, then each time you bake you can gradually increase the amount of whole-wheat flour.

If you want to go all the way towards your goal of optimal health, you can mill your own flour, introducing it into the diet in the same way.

Grinding your own grains ensures optimal nutrient content because the oils in grain start to break down and deteriorate within hours of being milled.

You can produce a finely ground flour with all its healthy oils, fiber, and nutrients by obtaining organic whole wheat berries from your local health food store or whole foods co-op. Or if you have the opportunity you might ask a local farmer about pesticide free grains.

To learn more about grinding your own flour, see the chapter on grain mills.

- **Easy Grains**

An easy way to prepare grains for breakfast is; before retiring for the night fill a wide mouth steel thermos with boiling water and let it stand for about ten minutes. Pour the water out of the thermos and pour in one cup of measured grain and fill the thermos with hot boiling water. Put the top on and leave overnight.

When you wake up you will have a hearty hot breakfast waiting for you. Drain any excess liquid.

You may want to add some chopped nuts, fresh or frozen fruit, butter, or honey for a satisfying nutritional breakfast.

Or if you're not a breakfast lover you could soak the grain overnight in hot broth, drain or leave soupy, then add sautéed onions and mushrooms or cooked carrots with butter, or other vegetables.

Another easy way to cook grains is by baking them in the oven. Rice is especially good prepared this way.

Combine one tablespoon of olive oil with two and one half cups of boiling water; add one cup of long grain brown rice and one teaspoon of sea salt. Cover and bake in a three hundred and fifty degree oven for about thirty-five minutes or until done. Fluff with a fork after ten minutes.

The crock-pot can also be used for cooking rice. One teaspoon of olive oil, one cup of uncooked converted long grain brown rice, two and a half cups of water and one teaspoon of salt.

Pour rice, water, and salt into greased slow cooker, cook on high two or three hours or until rice is tender, but not overcooked.

Cooked rice can be used in a variety of ways, as cereal or a quick snack, in puddings and custards, or added at the last minute to other dishes like soups and stews.

Brown rice has the husk and is healthier than white rice, which has its germ and fiber removed. The increased fiber in brown rice reduces fluctuations in blood sugar as opposed to white rice, which provokes an insulin reaction.

- **Amaranth**-is rich in lysine, calcium, phosphorus, and fiber, supplies all eight of the essential amino acids and is very high in protein. Although used as a grain, amaranth is actually a seed belonging to the pigweed family of plants. It has a pleasant flavor similar to fresh corn. The texture is somewhat like cream of wheat when boiled in water for making hot cereal, only creamier.

  Using two parts liquid to one part grain, add the amaranth to boiling water, reduce heat to lowest setting and simmer 25 minutes.

- **Barley-** Barley has been around since the Stone Age. When I think of barley my favorite soup from childhood comes to mind. While barley is good for thickening soups and stews it can be used for more than an addition to the soup or stew pot.

  It's most commonly known use is probably for making beer, and as an added ingredient in white flour for lighter fluffier baked goods. Barley is also used to make malted barley, or barley malt.

  Pearled barley is the most commonly found barley product available.

  Barley makes a delicious pilaf when cooked in chicken broth with onions and mushrooms.

  Barley flakes or whole grains make chewy breakfast cereal.

  When cooking with barley, use one cup of grain to three cups of liquid.

- **Bulgur**- Bulgur is toasted, steamed, dried kernels of wheat. It is easy to rehydrate, and to cook. The first thing I think of when

I see the word bulgur is Tabouli, a tasty grain salad.

Bulgur can be course, medium, finely ground, or pre-packaged with other ingredients added, and might say tabouli on the label. The medium grind is all-purpose and can be used for pilaf or tabouli salad. Use one cup of grain to two and a half cups of liquid. Cover, and cook on low heat twenty to twenty-five minutes.

- **Buckwheat-** is actually a seed from the rhubarb family of plants, contains all eight amino acids, and is very high in protein. The seeds are light brown in color and have a three-sided triangular shape.
- **Raw buckwheat** groats can be milled into flour that is excellent for making breads when used in addition to wheat flour, especially pancakes.
- **Roasted buckwheat** is known as kasha, which has a pleasant nut-like flavor. Kasha is a good substitute for rice pilaf.
    - **Soba noodles** from the Japanese are made with buckwheat flour and can be found in the international foods section of some grocery stores. They contain some wheat, so are not gluten free.

When cooking with buckwheat, if making kasha, which is roasted buckwheat groats (roasting keeps the grain from getting mushy) use one cup of buckwheat groats to two cups of liquid. Kasha is available in bulk at health food stores or co-ops.

For plain non-toasted buckwheat use one cup of raw buckwheat groats to five cups of liquid, bring to a boil on high, reduce heat to low, cover and cook ten to fifteen minutes.

Buckwheat pancakes from raw ground buckwheat groats are one of the most commonly made buckwheat products.

- **Cracked Wheat-**is whole kernels of wheat that have been cracked. The cooking time for cracked wheat can exceed two hours. My favorite method for cooking cracked wheat is the thermos method.

- **Kamut**- is an ancient form of wheat that originated in the fertile crescent of Egypt. The grains are large and have a kind of buttery flavor. It is available at health food stores.

- **Millet**- the millet most of us see is the kind used as birdseed. It is an excellent grain for people too.

Millet can be boiled like rice for breakfast and main dishes like pilaf, used for thickening and flavoring soups and stews, and added to flour when making bread. Use one cup of grain to three cups of water and cook for about forty-five minutes, or try an **easy grains** method (p156).

- **Steel Cut Oats** are steel cut whole oats sometimes called Scotch oats or Irish oats. They take considerably longer to cook than rolled oats. The thermos method produces chewy, creamy oats. To cook them the regular way use one cup of oats to two cups of boiling water, when they start to thicken reduce heat and simmer twenty minutes. Cover, let stand five minutes.

- **Old-fashioned rolled oats** are flattened flakes of whole oats. They take about eight minutes to cook. Combine one cup of old-fashioned rolled oats and two cups of cool water in a saucepan on medium low heat for five minutes stirring occasionally. Bring to a boil, remove from heat, cover, and let rest for approximately three minutes.

- **Quinoa**- an ancient grain originally from the Andes mountains, pronounced (keen-wah), is high in vitamins, contains all eight of the essential amino acids, and is very high in protein and calcium.

  The grains are naturally coated in saponins and must be thoroughly rinsed off before cooking.

  Place measured grains in a fine mesh strainer and set in a bowl of cool water, wash the grains thoroughly to remove the bitter saponins. Rinse and repeat.

  To cook combine one cup of grain with two and a half to three cups of water, bring to a boil, reduce heat to lowest setting, cover, and simmer for fifteen minutes.

  Quinoa flakes are now available and are quick and easy to prepare. Just stir into rapidly boiling water, stir and cook for ninety seconds, remove from heat and serve.

- **Spelt**- is a relative of wheat that is sometimes tolerated by those who are sensitive to wheat. It can be eaten as hot cereal; I prefer the easy grain thermos method for preparation. Spelt can be used in place of wheat flour for cooking and baking. It has less elasticity than wheat.

- **Teff**- an African cereal grain that yields a white flour when milled.

To cook the whole grain for hot cereal; use one cup of grain to three cups of water. Bring the water to a rapid boil, stir in the grain, reduce heat, cover, and simmer for twenty to thirty minutes.

All of the aforementioned grains can be ground for making hot cereals and a variety of different flours that contain all of their health giving properties when used right away.

Sourdough

The yeast breads of today are very different from the traditional yeast leavened breads they are derived from. Traditionally, yeast breads were started by capturing wild yeast to get a sponge that could be kept alive indefinitely by removing some of the sponge and adding fresh flour and water to it to feed the yeast. From start to finish it would take about three days to make a batch of bread. The starter could be kept going by feeding it to keep it alive.

Sourdough starter is available through health food stores or through the internet.

For a wild strain of your own starter: mix equal parts of fresh whole grain flour with lukewarm water, cover lightly, and set in a warm place for about twenty-four hours (in the oven with the light on or on top of the hot water heater). The mixture should bubble and foam and develop a slightly sour smell. If you see any dark brown or black mold on it throw it out.

To make bread add a cup of the starter to about four or five cups of fresh whole grain wheat flour and let rise in a warm place overnight. When it doubles in size and looks like a sponge, add four or five more cups of flour for the final rise, place in greased pans, and after it has risen, bake at 425* for twenty minutes to seal in the steam, reduce the heat to 375* and bake for another 45-50 minutes. You should now have a crusty chewy loaf of pleasantly sour bread. This bread will be heavier than fluffy store bought bread.

Sprouting Grains

Sprouting Grains is easy and increases the nutritional content of the grain. Any kind of clean organic seed can be used for sprouting. Make sure the seeds you use are for human consumption. (Never use garden seeds because they may contain fungicides or other chemicals).

Seeds for sprouting, and plastic canning jar tops with holes for straining are available through health food stores.

To get started you will need clean organic seeds, or grains, a quart size canning jar, a rubber band, and a piece of cheesecloth or plastic canning jar top, for air circulation and straining.

Begin by placing a couple of teaspoons of grain in the jar, cover with water and secure the top. If using cheesecloth secure it to the top of the jar with a rubber band. Soak overnight.

The next day; rinse the grain thoroughly and drain. Repeat the rinsing process two or three times more throughout the day and set the jar aside. Repeat for another day or two. When sprouts are about an inch long the process is complete and you can enjoy the benefits of sprouting.

Sprouts can be a source of green food by exposing them to sunlight. Just place the jar of sprouts in a sunny window for a few hours until they turn green. Rinse, drain, and refrigerate if not being used right away.

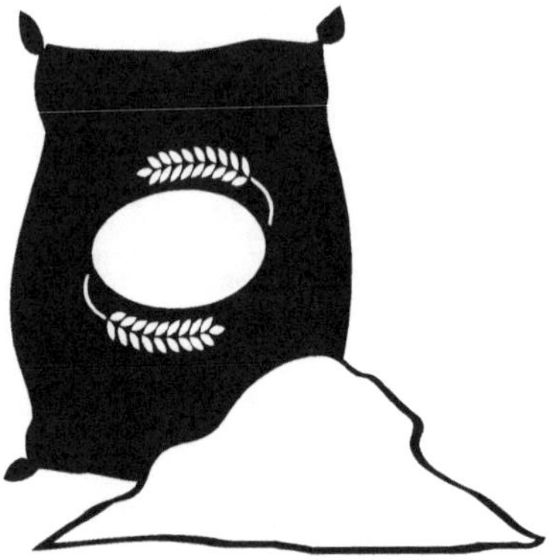

GRAIN MILLS

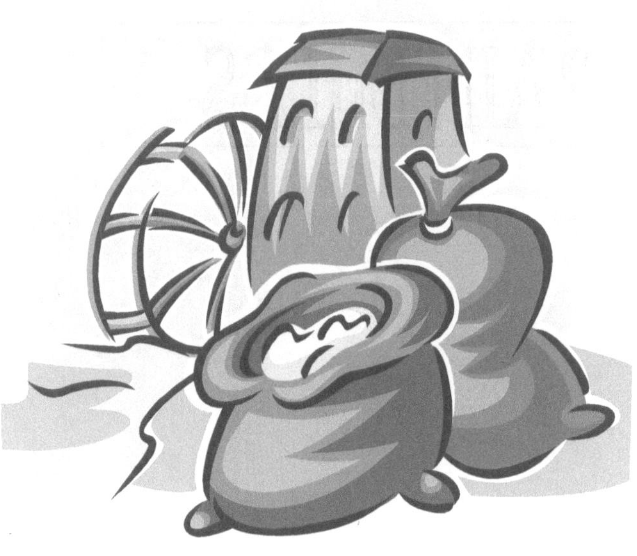

GRAIN MILLS

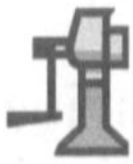

Grain mills can be used for more than just producing wheat flour. They can also be used for producing cereals like cream of wheat or rice, other kinds of whole grain cereals, and for obtaining nut flours. *(Hand operated mills may be preferable for grinding nuts).*

Right now you might be thinking about how you can buy cereals like cream of wheat or cream of rice and flours already ground up from the grocery store.

While that is true, it is also true that soon after it is ground, the store product will have lost most of it's nutritional properties, and therefore is a lesser quality product than fresh milled cereals, or flours, no matter which grain is used.

With all the different grains available, grinding whole grains yourself allows for greater variety and nutrients.

You can produce finely ground whole-grain flour using a hand mill. Begin by grinding a coarse meal and repeat reducing to a finer texture until the desired results are achieved. Three passes should be sufficient to acquire finely ground flour. Begin with a course meal and adjust the setting after each pass to make grinding easier until the desired result is achieved.

For large quantities of flour you may prefer an electric motorized mill. Not all mills are created equal. There are some excellent products on the market, and it pays to do the research required before making an investment.

If you are planning on using the mill for grinding nuts a hand mill is preferable.

I have a friend who bought a top of the line motorized grain mill, which produced an excellent finely ground whole grain flour from whole-wheat berries. When she was thinking about selling it I asked her if the mill could be used for grinding nuts and she said no because of moisture or maybe the higher content of natural oils contained in the nuts.

My preferred grain mill for grinding nuts into nut flours is the Corona hand mill that I had on hand from when I was previously using it for grinding grains into flours and meal. It can easily be disassembled and put in the dishwasher.

At the time of this writing, a similar mill is available through the internet from www.northerntool.com for $14.99 plus shipping.

To order by phone: 1-800-221-0516 or (952-895-6866)

NUT FLOURS

Primary Concerns by Sherry Ferrell

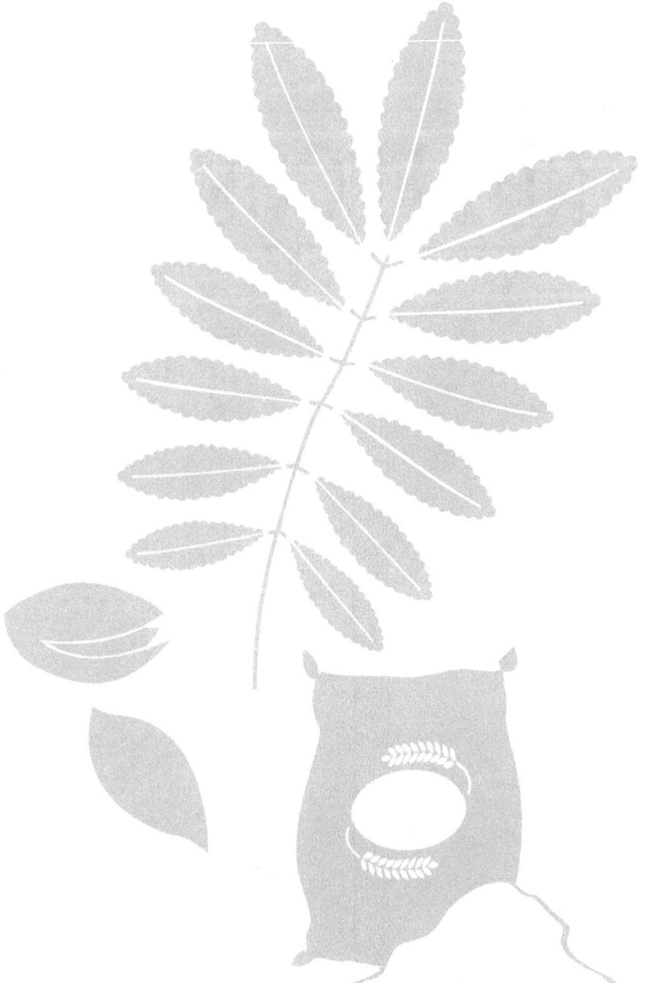

NUT FLOURS

A food processor can be used to make a coarse meal, or for making nut butters, which will occur if the grinding time for meal is exceeded.

For a fine-textured nut flour a hand operated mill is the best tool for the job. Almonds are a little harder to grind than pecans or walnuts. Using sliced almonds or coarsely chopping whole almonds before hand grinding will make the job quicker and easier. For most recipes one or two cups of nuts is all that is required. A one-pound bag of sliced almonds equals five and one-third cups. Currently the cost per cup averages under a dollar.

A pound or two of nuts can be kept at room temperature if they are going to be used relatively soon.

Nuts and nut flour are available in bulk through the Internet @www.truefoodsmarket.com. However the cost is considerably higher than buying nuts from a wholesale buying club and grinding them into flour yourself. When ordering from the True Foods Market website, click on nuts and seeds, then when the nuts and seeds page comes up, click on nut flours and meals, on the next page click on food & nutrition.

Storing nuts in the refrigerator or freezer if they are not going to be used right away can extend the shelf life.

A cup of raw whole almonds will yield about one cup of finely ground almond flour.

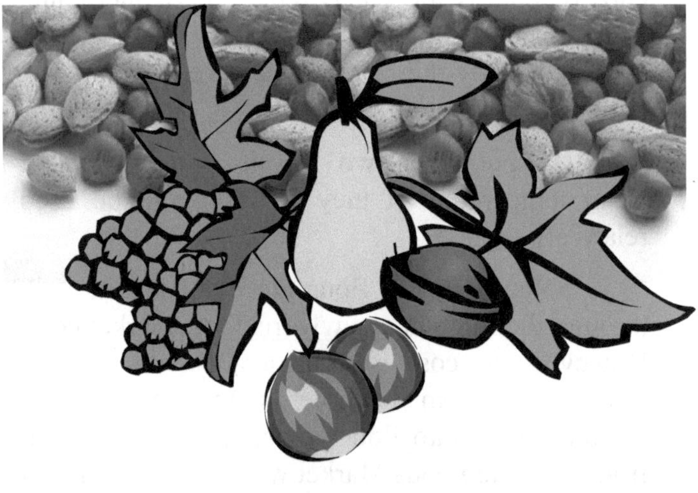

MICROWAVES

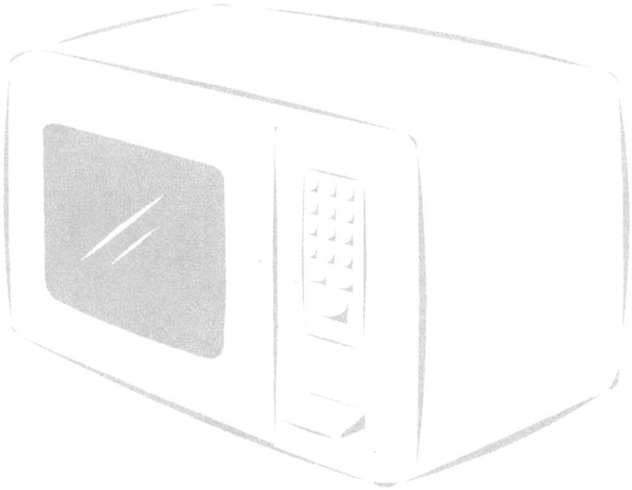

MICROWAVE COOKING

I have researched and found no definitive answers for or against the use of microwaves for cooking. I have read a few articles opposing the use of microwaves, and I believe the evidence shown was based on use that was out of context with ordinary microwave cooking.

Traditional cooking methods are preferable for cooking meats. The heat in microwaves tends to be uneven and there is always the possibility that bacteria could be present in undercooked areas.

The use of plastics and paper in microwaves introduces the possibility of chemicals leaching into food; therefore it is safer to use glass cookware.

My nutritionist states emphatically that one may as well eat cardboard because anything cooked in the microwave comes out depleted. That being a possibility gives me pause for using the microwave for cooking.

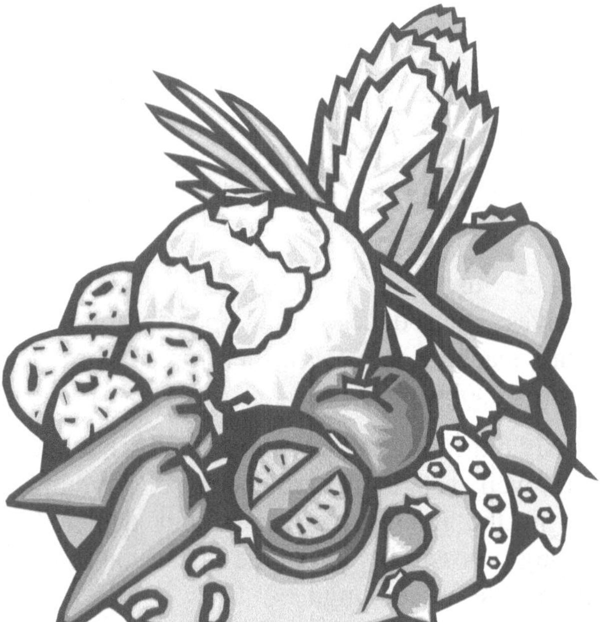

JUICING

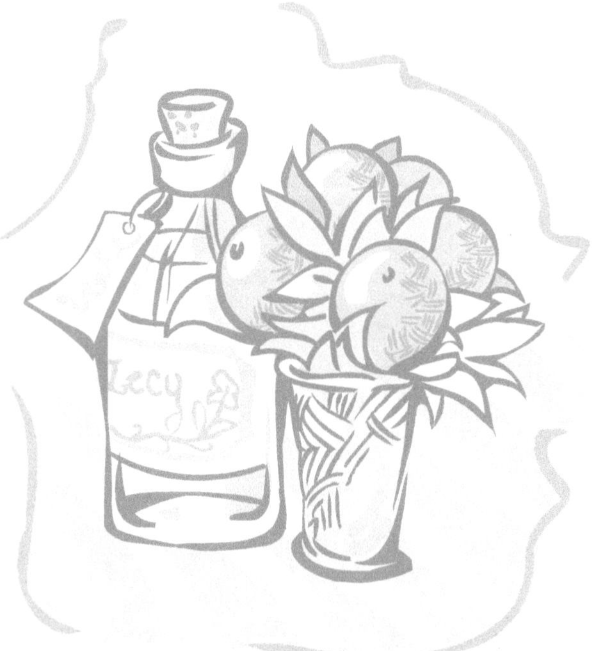

JUICING

My first encounter with fresh juices other than orange juice or lemonade was an eye opening experience. The flavors were unique and satisfying and my energy level increased and was sustained far longer than I expected. My interest peaked and I invested in a juice machine and a book about juicing and it's many benefits.

Fresh juices contain enzymes that aid digestion and nutrients that support the body's ability to heal itself.

I used to make fresh juice and throw away the pulp that was left over. Now I use the pulp and add other ingredients like ground up seeds or nuts, olive oil, flaxseed oil, or walnut oil. Sometimes I add herbs, depending on what my needs are at the time.

Following is an example of one of my favorite juices.

4 large carrots, peeled

1 coin sized piece of fresh ginger, peeled

1 apple washed, cored and cut into eighths

This juice is sweet and warming. The pulp is good with a little bit of honey, cinnamon and chopped walnuts, or as a salad with olive oil, sea salt, and fresh lemon juice. (2 Servings)

Listed below are some books on juicing by various authors.

- **Juicing for Life** by Cherie Calbom and Maureen Keane
- **Juiceman's Power of Juicing** by Jay Kordich
- **The Book Of Raw Fruit and Vegetable Juices and Drinks** by William H. Lee R.Ph., Ph. D.

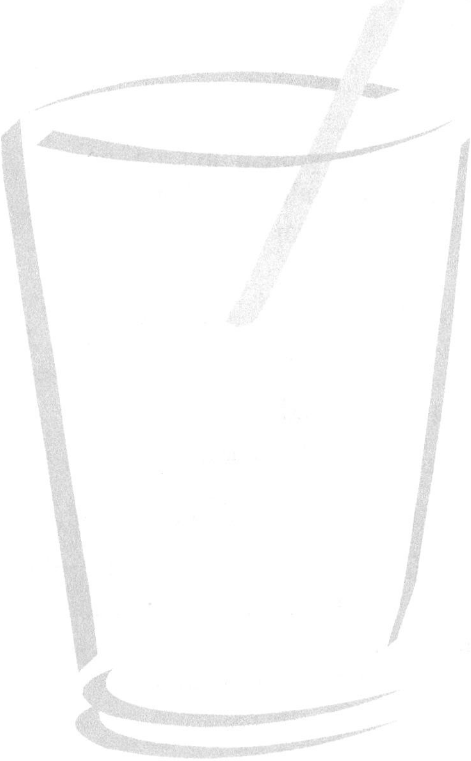

HERB CLOSET

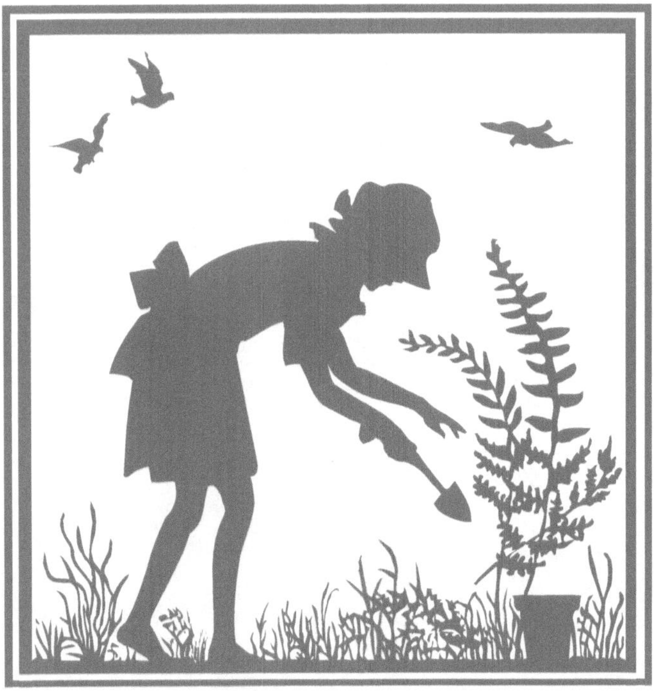

HERB CLOSET

Many of us use herbs for adding flavor and variety to meals during cooking and baking. Basil is the primary ingredient used to make pesto, sage is used in poultry seasoning, and ginger and garlic add flavor to many dishes. Herbs also have practical value as part of the home medicine cabinet.

A long time ago the medicine cabinet at my house gave way to the herb closet. Just as many of us keep a first aid kit for emergencies, I have learned to keep herbs on hand for the same reason. After trying different herbs for common health concerns I found that many were good to have on hand at all times.

Following is a list of the herbs we use most often. Follow product recommendations.

- **Arnica**- very effective for bruises, and muscle pain and stiffness associated with strain or overexertion. Available as a cream or gel for topical use, homeopathically for sublingual use and as a tincture for trauma. (Arnica should not be used on broken skin as it can cause blisters).

- **Calendula**- used for sunburns, chafing, cuts, scrapes, and open sores. Calendula is soothing, initiates rapid healing, and is antibacterial and antifungal. The dried flower petals can be used to make tea, which is useful for applying to minor skin conditions such as diaper rash, cuts, scrapes, and burns. (Calendula cream is especially soothing for irritation related to yeast infection). Also available as a tincture, cream, or gel.
- **Chamomile**- calming, relieves pain, good for colic, teething, upset stomach, fever, and restlessness in children. (Avoid if sensitive to ragweed. Daily use can lead to ragweed allergy). Chamomile herb tea and homeopathic chamomilla have similar uses.

- **Cinnamon-** warming, relieves colds and congestion, improves energy, aids digestion, relieves diarrhea and nausea.

- **Clove-** ground up cloves ease toothache and mouth pain.

- **Echinacea-** immune enhancing, reduces inflammation. Especially useful for colds, flu, and urinary tract infections. (Avoid if sensitive to ragweed or sunflowers). Goldenseal, and Oregon grape are also natural antibiotics.

- **Elderberry-** Used for colds, and flu. Prevents viruses from replicating. Reduces flu symptoms. Shortens duration. Available in vitamin and herb shops. Elderberry is the primary ingredient in Sambucol, a cold and flu remedy for children.

- **Garlic-** natural antibiotic, blood purifier, aids digestion. I have used garlic successfully for ringing ears and wart removal (p57-58). Garlic body odor is a common side effect of taking pure garlic. Odorless supplements are available.

- **Ginger**- antihistamine, warming, promotes perspiration, useful for colds and sore throat, nausea, and cramps. Helps expel gas. Ginger can be combined with other herbs to enhance their beneficial properties. (Avoid if you have gastritis or peptic ulcer).

- **Goldenseal-** fights infection, immune enhancing, can cause nausea or vomiting in sensitive individuals. (Should not be used while breastfeeding)

- **Oregon Grape Root-** related to barberry, fights infection. (Should not be used while breastfeeding)

- **Peppermint**-Tea is soothing, cooling, strengthening, and relieves pain. Aids digestion, increases stomach acid. Useful for colds, fevers, headaches.

- **Red Raspberry leaf**- makes good tea, iced or hot. Good for sore throats, valued as a treatment for diarrhea. Women have used red raspberry leaf tea for centuries to tone the uterus. Helps reverse urinary incontinence.

St. John's Wort- invaluable in the treatment of crush injuries such as having had fingers shut in a door. I keep an olive oil based extract and an alcohol based tincture on hand for crush injuries and bruises with broken skin. Add a few drops of either preparation to about 1/3 cup of warm water and soak for ten to fifteen minutes. (st. john's wort can cause sunlight sensitivity in some people, if a rash develops discontinue use).

Witch Hazel- available at pharmacies and some grocery stores, witch hazel is effective when applied externally to sprains, strains, hemorrhoids, insect bites and stings. For hemorrhoids soak a piece of gauze with witch hazel and tuck into affected area.

Primary Concerns by Sherry Ferrell

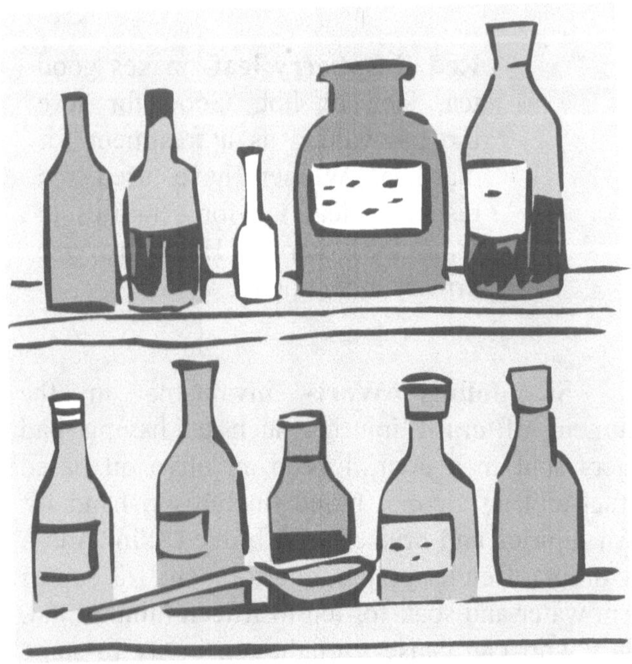

RECIPES

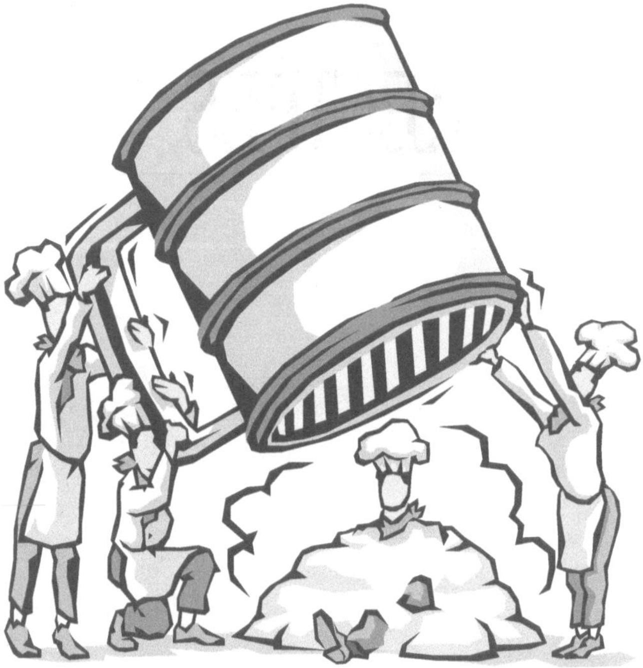

RECIPES

When making baked goods I use almond flour and pasteurized powdered egg whites *(I buy in bulk from a whole foods co-op)* to help with binding, texture and rising. Hand mixing is sufficient because almond flour is much lighter than flours made from grains. Almond flour can be used in equal measure in place of all purpose white flour in most baked goods recipes.

When grinding almonds to make almond flour one cup of almonds yields about one cup of almond flour. *(Sliced or chopped almonds are easier to grind than whole almonds)* Store any leftover almond flour in the refrigerator.

For the recipes

c = cup t = teaspoon T = tablespoon
* = Degrees Fahrenheit

Lightly grease measuring cup before measuring honey, to prevent sticking.

These recipes use very few convenience food items because I hardly ever use them. I have been cooking this way for about five years and have found it increasingly easier to use fresh ingredients in my recipes. Most people would see that as a huge inconvenience but I find the over-all improvement in my quality of life has been worth the extra effort it takes.

Almond Milk

Almond milk is commercially available but usually sweetened with either sugar (cane juice) or brown rice syrup. I prefer homemade almond milk rather than store bought. Almond milk can replace cows milk in recipes. Following are two versions. The first is creamy and strained for drinking; the second is unstrained and quick.

A fine mesh coffee filter will be needed for the first recipe to separate the pulp from the milk. The filter is top rack dishwasher safe.

This recipe starts with whole almonds, which will need to be blanched to make the milk sweeter and creamier. You can use store bought blanched almonds, but blanching your own almonds is economical. (If starting with store bought blanched almonds skip this step). Hot, but not boiled, water helps make the milk creamier without affecting the enzymes in the nuts.

2c. boiled water 1c. whole almonds 2 c. hot, but not boiled, water 1c. ice 1 c. cool water to chill

Soak almonds in boiled water off heat for 2 minutes. Drain and cover with cool water, place an almond between thumb and forefinger and squeeze allowing the almond to slip from its skin. Repeat until all the almonds are peeled.

Place the peeled almonds in a blender with 2 c. hot but not boiled water and blend until milky white and the pulp is fine-textured. Place coffee filter in another strainer and set them both to rest over a 2qt. Saucepan or ½ gallon pitcher. Pour blended almond milk into mesh coffee filter and let it rest until the milk has run through the pulp.

To the milk add 1 T. honey and 1 ½ t. vanilla if desired. Add 1 c. cool water and 1 c. ice to chill, or 2 c. cool water. Makes four cups Almond Milk.

Easy Almond Milk

This recipe is less creamy than the one above it, but good for cooking and baking, making smoothies, or for pouring over "Easy Breakfast" (page *198),* or fresh fruit.

1 c pure water ¼ c sliced almonds 1t honey

Place water, almonds and honey in a deep container (2 quart pitcher) and blend with a stick blender.

Ginger Tea

Mince 1 one-inch piece of fresh ginger *(a heavy duty garlic press works great for this)* and put in a coffee cup. Cover with eight to twelve ounces of pure boiling water. Steep 3-5 minutes, add honey to taste.

For variation: Add a bag of chamomile tea before covering with water.

Almond Banana Smoothie This recipe satisfies the need for a special treat.

½ c almond milk ½ t vanilla extract 1 t honey

1 medium banana

Combine in blender on high speed until thick.

For a frozen treat place mixture in freezer until firm and enjoy!

Easy Breakfast

Place 1/4 c sliced almonds, chopped walnuts, or pecans in a cereal bowl, drizzle with honey, add some fresh or frozen fruit, cover with cold water, apple juice, or almond milk.

Orange-Jewel

This recipe is a spin on an old favorite, kind of like a snow cone. An ice shaver is required if you want the snow cone similarity. It can be made in the blender with ice for a frozen drink instead of a snow cone.

Shave ice and pack it with your hands fitting it into two small or one large glass Squeeze juice from 2 medium sized oranges and stir 1 or 2 drops peppermint extract into juice, and pour over shaved ice.

Makes 2 small or 1 large orange jewel.

For the blender version: place several ice cubes in the blender with the juice and peppermint extract. Blend on high until slushy.

Peaches 'N' Cream Casserole

This recipe was adapted from one of my favorite recipe books Lean And Luscious and Meatless Volume 3 in the Lean and Luscious series by Bobbie Hinman and Millie Snyder. The original recipe calls for oats and milk, which are off limits for me so I adapted it, using quinoa and apple juice. Any peachy type of fruit can be used such as mangoes or nectarines. **(Recipe begins here and continues on the next page)**

¾ c Quinoa flakes ¾ c thinly sliced fresh or frozen peaches

2 T honey 2 t egg white powder 1 t vanilla
1 /8 t almond extract 1 ½ c apple juice

Place the quinoa flakes and egg white powder in a medium sized mixing bowl and stir together with a whisk until lumps in egg white powder disappear. Add all other ingredients, stir together, and pour into a greased 1-quart casserole dish. Bake on 350* for 40-50 minutes.

Orange Blueberry Breakfast

1 orange, peeled, sectioned, and cut into chunks. Sprinkled with unsweetened coconut, fresh or frozen blueberries, and toasted almonds, pecans, or both. Drizzle with a thin stream of honey and serve.

Honey-'N'-Cinnamon Apples

Peel core and slice an apple, arrange slices in a cereal bowl. Add cinnamon, drizzle with honey and top with raw or toasted walnut, almond, or pecan pieces.

Sweet Potato Treat

Peel and mash a hot or cold baked sweet potato and top with a small amount of drizzled honey, sprinkle on some cinnamon and raw or toasted chopped nuts.

Low-Sugar Jelly- This is really a fruit spread we use in place of store bought jelly. Mash fruit and strain excess juice, add a little bit of honey. Good on nut flour bread or spread on a banana. For orange marmalade zest a little rind before peeling, section the fruit, combine fruit, rind, and honey.

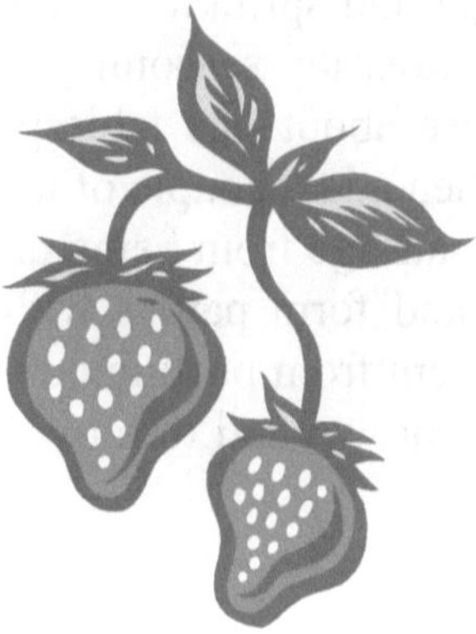

Scrambled Eggs

Adding water to eggs makes them light and fluffy. Add 1-2 Tablespoons of water to two eggs and beat until light yellow in color. Season to taste, cook on medium heat stirring occasionally until cooked through.

Sausage-Homemade sausage is easy to make and preferable to prepared products containing unwanted ingredients. Dry rubs work well for seasoning meats.

Start with one pound of fresh ground pork or other meat and sprinkle in some salt and pepper or your favorite seasoning. (I like sage and usually use about one tablespoon per pound of meat). Then add a couple of tablespoons of oil to keep the sausage from being dry. Mix everything together and form patties with indented centers to keep them from puffing out. Cook on medium high until brown and turn over. Brown the other side.

ENCHILADAS

1 chopped pepper, any color 1 c water
1-pound ground chicken 1 onion, chopped
1 small can tomato paste
1 heaping T oregano 1 heaping T cumin

Brown chicken and set aside. Sauté chopped peppers and onions until tender; add seasonings, tomato paste, and water and cook on medium until heated through. Add chicken, and stir together.

5x chili mix

Can be used for dry rub on ribs and chicken wings or for just plain chili. This recipe can be reduced, but we use it so often we make it up large.

½ c. onion powder 3 T. chili powder 1 t. salt

1t. cayenne 2 T. cumin

Combine all ingredients and store in an airtight container.

Ribs

Coat any style pork ribs with a thin layer of olive oil and sprinkle a couple of handfuls of 5x chili mix over both sides, rub it in, and bake on 425* for 20 minutes coat in very thinly drizzled honey. Bake for ten or fifteen minutes more.

We usually use a half rack of ribs. If the quantity gets too large they don't caramelize as well.

Venison Ribs

Preheat oven to 425*. Coat ribs with a generous amount of olive oil and rub dried sage all over both sides. Bake for approximately 30 minutes.

Crock-Pot Chicken

This is a great evening meal at the end of a busy day.

Place one large roasting chicken in crock-pot and cook on high 3-4 hours or on low for 7-8 hours. Add a salad, sliced tomatoes or cucumbers, and steamed veggies for a quick satisfying meal.

Spicy Crock-Pot Chicken

This spicy recipe is popular at my house and rarely results in leftovers.

2 t salt 2 t paprika ½ t cayenne 1 T onion powder ½ t black pepper

Combine spices and rub mixture over one large roasting chicken. Place some of the mixture inside the cavity of the chicken. Cook in crock-pot on **high 3-4 hours**

Chicken wings

Place wings in a large bowl, drizzle with olive oil and sprinkle on a couple of handfuls of 5x chili mix (p.203). Stir to coat, scoop wings from the bowl into a large roasting pan. Bake at 375* for 40 minutes. If you like them sweet and caramelized, drizzle on a thin stream of honey the last ten minutes of cooking time.

5x Chili

1 lb. ground meat (*beef, chicken, or pork*) ¼ c. 5x chili mix, 3 large tomatoes peeled, cored, and chopped. 1 large onion, chopped 1 large green pepper, chopped

Brown meat with 5x chili mix (p.203), set aside, and sauté the chopped onion, green pepper, and tomatoes. Cook until onions are translucent. Combine all ingredients, stir together and enjoy!

Spicy Chicken Strips

1 pound boneless chicken strips Mix together 2 t salt 2 t paprika ½ t cayenne 1 T onion powder ½ t black pepper

Coat strips in olive oil and sprinkle with spice mixture, cook on medium high heat until slightly brown and tender.

Dilled Chicken Spread

1 c. of shredded cooked chicken dash pepper ¼ c. mayonnaise ¼ t. Onion powder 2 t. Prepared mustard ¼ t. Dried dill

Combine and stir together. Good for stuffing tomatoes, celery, or cucumbers.

Chicken Stir-Fry

1 cooked chicken breast chopped 1 lb frozen stir-fry vegetables 1 one-inch chunk fresh ginger 8 slices of frozen peaches thawed 1 T honey

Cook frozen stir-fry vegetables. Add ginger by slicing and pressing it through a heavy-duty garlic press over the vegetables. Run the blade of a paring knife over the ginger as it comes through the press. Mash thawed peach sections, drain and stir in honey. Add to other ingredients, toss, and serve.

Quick-N-Easy Chicken Ginger Soup

This recipe, which begins here and continues on the next page is one of my favorites. The ginger is warming and the bag salad makes it very easy to prepare.

Combine two cups of chicken broth *(I save the broth from crock pot cooked chicken)* with two cups of chopped chicken and one cup of fresh carrots, thinly sliced. Cook on high for about ten minutes, or until boiling. Stir and add two cups of fresh salad, like the kind you use for tossed salads, turn off heat, and cover. Let rest for about three minutes, or until lettuce wilts. Add a one-inch piece of finely chopped ginger. (*or slice four or five nickel size pieces of ginger and squeeze them one at a time through a heavy duty garlic press directly into the soup, slicing the ginger as it comes through the press*). Stir ginger into soup and enjoy!

Bacon Topped Tomatoes

Wash and dry a large tomato, slice the bottom off and dispose of it. Slice the top and outer walls into five sections, remove seeds and set aside. Remove seeds from center core and divide core into five or six slices. Top each tomato section with the following bacon mixture.

2 T Mayonnaise 1 T Real Bacon Bits ¼ t Onion powder

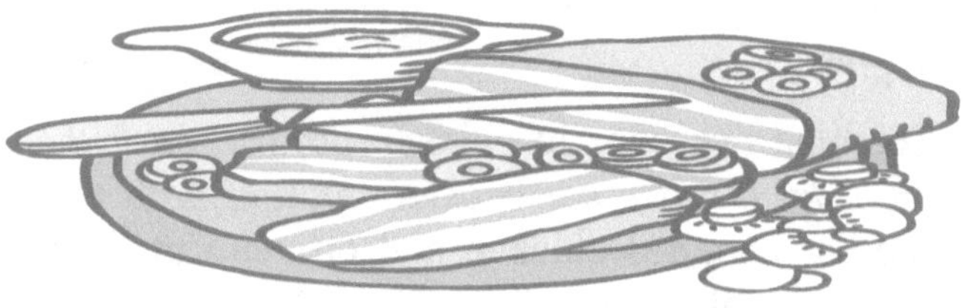

Roasted Yellow Squash or Zucchini

Two Medium Yellow Squash or Zucchini
Olive oil

Oregano, Thyme, or Basil   Salt & Pepper

Cut squash diagonally into ½ inch slices and place in a large bowl. Drizzle with olive oil, stir and season.

Place on a baking sheet and bake at 375* for 15-20 minutes. Turn slices over and bake for an additional 15-20 minutes.

Roasting enhances the flavor of these vegetables. This recipe is sure to please even those who think they don't like squash!

Roasted Tomato

Peel, core, seed, and section a medium sized tomato. Sprinkle with olive oil and basil, or Worcestershire sauce, and bake at 425* for 30 minutes.

Peas-Onions-and Mushrooms

1 lb of fresh or frozen peas 1 bunch of scallions sliced

½ lb of fresh button mushrooms sliced ¼ c water

Pour water into a two-quart saucepan, cover and bring to a boil, add the other ingredients and cook on medium 10-15 minutes or until the peas are tender. Drain and sprinkle with salt and pepper.

Spinach with Onions

This is a favorite at my house.

1 lb of fresh or frozen spinach 1 medium onion

Cut the onion up, sauté, and set-aside. Cook spinach till wilted or heated through, add sautéed onions, stir together, and serve.

Tangy Beets

Most of the foods we eat contribute to an over acid state. Lemons have an alkalizing effect on the body (for more on lemons see p122). Vinegar is usually made from corn unless it is red wine or apple cider vinegar. Commercial vinegars are usually distilled. When using vinegar my preference is Bragg's raw unfiltered organic apple cider vinegar, available at health food stores, and some herb shops.

1 16oz. Can of beets with liquid   2 fresh lemons or ½ c. vinegar   ¼ c. honey

Juice lemons and combine them with the beets and honey in a medium saucepan. Bring to a boil turn heat off cover and let stand 5-10 minutes. Chill or eat warm, whatever your preference. Chilling overnight increases the flavor.

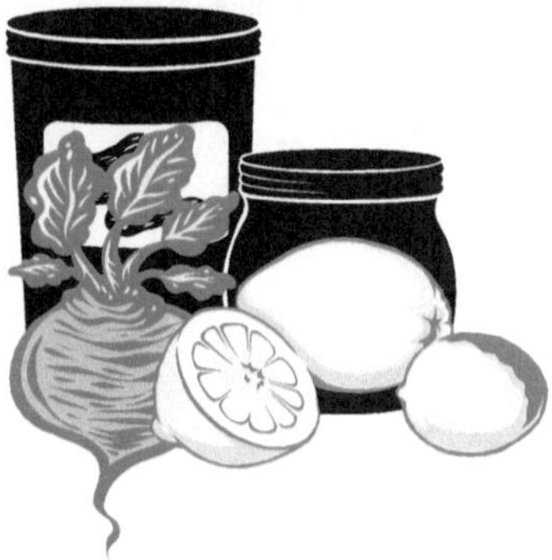

Carrot Salad

Peel a carrot and discard the peelings. Using the peeling tool shave wide thin strips of carrot into a salad bowl. Top with your favorite salad dressing.

Rosemary Roasted vegetables

Preheat oven to 425*

1 large zucchini cut lengthwise into fourths, then cut into large chunks lg handful cherry tomatoes ½ lb sliced mushrooms

Place in a large bowl, drizzle with olive oil and sprinkle with fresh or dried rosemary, salt and pepper. Stir together, spread on baking sheet and bake for 20-30 minutes.

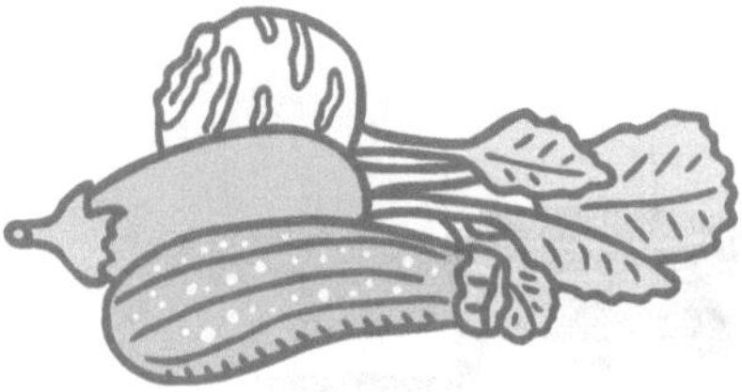

Maple Nut Cookies Preheat oven to 325*

3 c almond flour ½ c chopped nuts 1 egg ¾ t baking soda 1t water ½ c oil 1/3 c maple syrup pinch of salt

Stir all ingredients together, form 1½-inch balls, flatten on cookie sheet. Bake for 15-20 minutes.

Variation:

For a small batch of Maple Nut Cookies that can be baked in the toaster oven. Preheat oven to 325*

¾ c Almond flour 2 T Butter ½ a beaten egg ¼ t baking soda

2 T maple syrup pinch of salt 2 T chopped nuts

Drop dough by tablespoons on a cookie sheet and bake for 15-20 minutes.

Shortbread Preheat oven to 325*

¾ c butter (I use Smart Balance non hydrogenated spread)

1/3 c honey 3 c almond flour 2 t vanilla extract

¼ t almond extract ¼ t cardamom

Cream butter and honey, add vanilla, almond extract, blend and add dry ingredients, press into an eight inch pan and bake for 30-40 minutes.

Chocolate Chip Cookies Preheat oven to 325*

3 c almond flour ½ c chocolate chips ½ c chopped nuts 1 egg ¾ t baking soda 1t water ½ c oil

1/3 c honey pinch of salt

Stir all ingredients together, form 1½-inch balls, flatten on cookie sheet. Bake for 15-20 minutes. These disappear fast around our house.

Variation: For a small batch of Chocolate chip cookies that can be baked in the toaster oven. Preheat toaster oven to 325*

¾ c Almond flour 2 T Butter ½ a beaten egg ¼ t baking soda

2 T honey pinch of salt 2 T chocolate chips 2 T nuts

Stir all ingredients together, form 1½-inch balls, flatten on cookie sheet. Bake for 15-20 minutes.

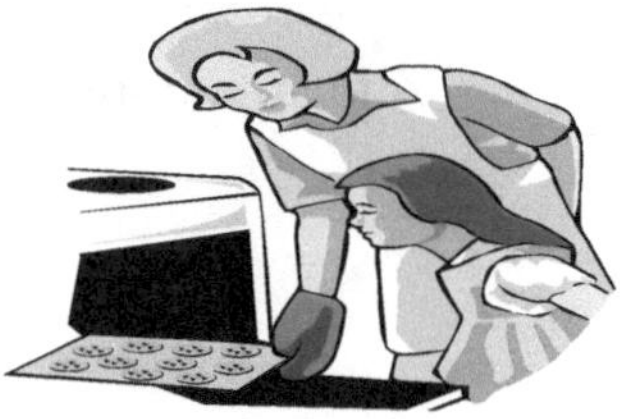

Carrot Cake Preheat oven to 325* 8" baking pan

1 c almond flour ½ t cinnamon 4 t egg white powder ¼ t baking soda 1½ c finely shredded carrot 5 T honey

Mix dry ingredients, add wet ingredients and stir together. Bake 30-40 minutes.

Variation:

Replace shredded carrots with a raw, finely shredded sweet potato. Just peel the sweet potato (as you would a normal everyday white potato), before shredding.

Variation: Replace carrots with shredded apple. Wash apple, dry, core, and shred.

Topping:

In a small bowl, mix one tablespoon of honey with **1/16** t of vanilla, orange or lemon extract. Lightly grease the spoon before stirring to keep the honey from sticking. Drizzle in small streams over top of cake.

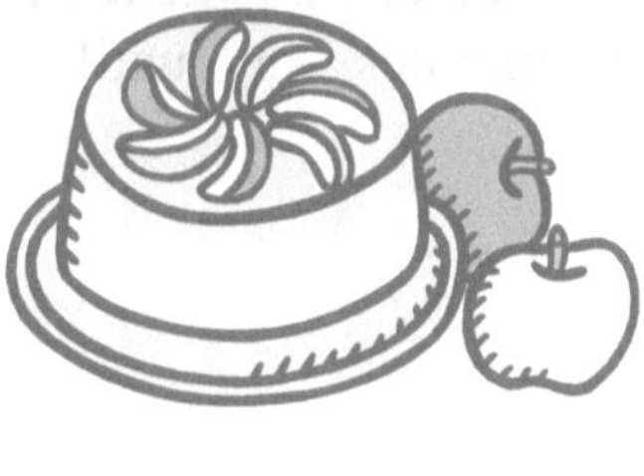

Mini Apple Muffin Recipe Preheat oven to 325*

1c almond flour 4 t egg white powder ¼ t Baking Soda ¼ c finely chopped apple ¼ c honey 1 tsp vanilla

1/4 c unsweetened applesauce

Line mini muffin pan with mini baking cups, combine dry ingredients, sift, then stir together in mixing bowl. Add all other ingredients, stir together and spoon into individual baking cups. Bake 30 minutes. Test for being done by poking a toothpick in the center of a muffin.

"Apple Pie"

Peel core and slice an apple, then top with cinnamon, drizzled honey, and walnut, almond, or pecan pieces. *(The nuts are a healthy replacement for traditional piecrust).* For more than one serving increase the number of apples and proceed with the other ingredients. Bake at 350* for 20-30 minutes or until tender.

Lemon-Poppyseed Cake Preheat oven to 325*.

1c almond flour 4t egg white powder
¼ t baking soda ½ t. baking powder
1T poppyseeds 1T lemon oil

¼ c honey 1T water

Combine dry ingredients, sift, stir together, add all other ingredients, mix well. *Lemon oil is available at gourmet shops. I like the flavor better than lemon extract in this recipe. However, if you don't have any lemon oil then use 1 T vegetable oil and 1 ½ tsp. lemon extract.

Pour into a greased ovenproof cereal bowl, like Pyrex or Corning Ware. Bake for 35 minutes.

Test for being done by poking a toothpick through the center. For a larger cake, double the recipe and bake in a greased eight-inch cake pan and add 7-10 minutes to the baking time.

Variation: Lemon Cranberry cake
Add 2 T chopped fresh or frozen cranberries instead of the poppyseeds.

Almond Milk Frozen Blueberry Treat

We like this best with homemade almond milk.

Place a handful of frozen blueberries in a cereal bowl and cover with chilled almond milk. Drizzle with honey. The frozen blueberries clump together with the almond milk. Yum!

FROZEN FRUIT CHOCOLATE

This recipe requires a blender.

1 medium frozen banana cut into slices 5 frozen strawberries 1½ T frozen orange concentrate
1 t Watkins chocolate extract
1 t vanilla extract 2 T olive oil 1 T honey
Water

Put first seven ingredients in blender and pulse on high adding water until the mixture resembles a smoothie. Pour into a container, cover, and freeze. To increase fiber and protein counts add 1/3 c sliced almonds and two heaping tablespoons of egg white powder. Blend on high for about 30 seconds. Pour into a tall glass. Enjoy!

Strawberry Banana Smoothie This recipe requires a blender.

1 lg banana 5-6 frozen strawberries
½ c water 2 T almonds

Peel banana, place all ingredients in blender, and blend on high until smooth. Enjoy!

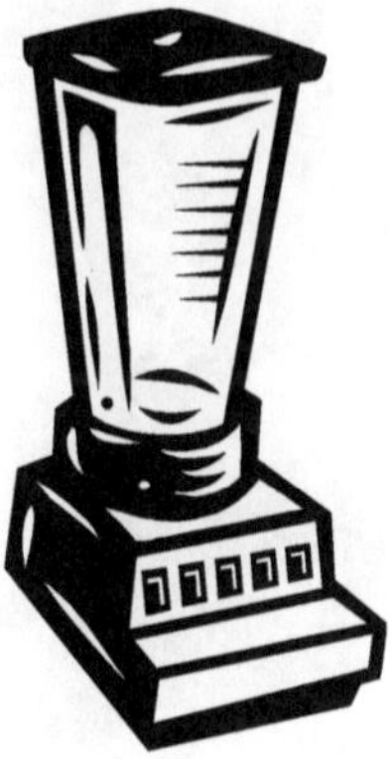

Index

Contact Information

e-mail sherryferrell@fersherpublishing.com

Mailing address :
Sherry Ferrell
P. O. Box 2762
Chester, Va 23831

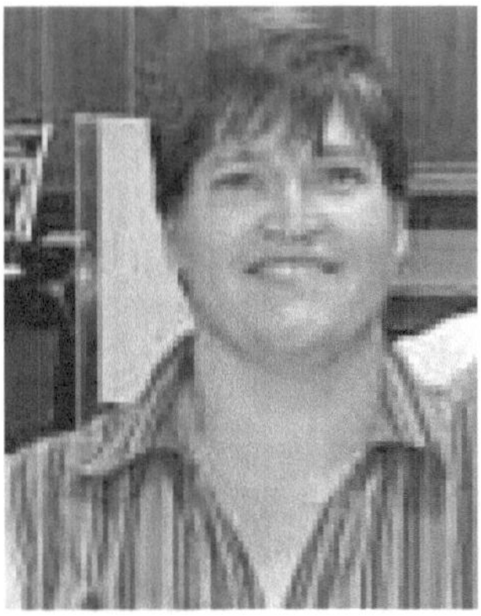

Sherry Ferrell resides with her family in Richmond, Virginia.

Made in United States
Troutdale, OR
11/03/2026

56852549R00130